HABITS FOR NURSES

AN INJECTION OF SIMPLICITY IN A STAT WORLD

BEAU SALTS, RN, B.S.

Copyright © 2020

All rights reserved. No part of this guide may be reproduced in any form without permission in writing from the author except in the case of brief quotations embodied in critical articles or reviews.

CONTENTS

Introduction 1
Mental Strategies 7
  Rituals 7
    Morning Routine: 8
    Mid-Day Routine: 9
    Night-Time Routine: 10
  Self-Improvement 2020 12
  Momentum 14
    Momentum – Take Action 16
  Influences 17
  Control Your Thoughts 18
  Addiction 21
    How to Fight Back 25
  Keep Calm 32
    Meet Maximus 34
    Squeeze 39
  Sleep 39
    Meditate Before Sleeping 41
    Diffuse Lavender Essential Oils 41
    Turn Down the Temperature in Your Bedroom .41
    Sleep in a Completely Dark Room 42
Emotional Strategies 43
  Communications 43
    Bedside Manner 43
    How to Handle the Workplace Bully 47
    Managing the Perfect Patient 52

    Handling Patients Going Through Hard Times 53
    Protecting Yourself in All Situations 54
Inner Strength 57
Indulge in humor 59
Faith 61
Self-Compassion 63
    Practice Self-Encouragement 64
    Do Recreational Activities 64
    Write Your Feelings Down Honestly 65
    Practice Mindfulness 65
Meditation 65
    Simple Meditation Technique 66
Pets (Not Your Spouse) 68
Hobbies and Free Time 70
    Do Something That Interests You 72
    Do Something That Challenges You 72
    Set Goals for Yourself 72
    Try Merging Your Goals if Possible 73

Physical Health Strategies 75
Watch Your Back 75
    Herniated Discs 77
    Inversion Plan of Action 85
    Proactive Back Health 89
    Instant Relief 93
Workouts for the Time-Impaired Nurse 95
    Home Gym 98
    How to Workout 100
    The Nurse Workout 105
    Post-Workout Stretching 114
    The Impossibly Busy Nurse's Workout 114
Considerations for Nightshift Nurses 117
    Get Enough Sleep 118

  Make Healthy Nutritional Choices 119
  Take Time to Exercise 119
  Bond with Your Colleagues 120
  Maintain a Healthy Lifestyle Outside of Work .. 120
  Monitor Vitamin D Level 120
  Use Light Therapy 121
 Snack and Lunch Options 121
 Hydration 124
 Caffeine 126
 Apps 127

Organizational Strategies 129
 Career Development 129
  On-The-Job Organization 129
  Habits 133
  Maintain and Expand Your Knowledge 136
 Finances 140
  Fuel 144
 Recurrent Chores – Laundry Edition 147
  Store It Dirty 149
  Store It Clean 153
  Revisiting Delegation 158
 The Logistics of Lunch 162

Afterword 167

About the Author 171

Appendix 1: Recommended Products 173

Appendix 2: Resources By Chapter 177
 Mental Strategies 177
 Emotional Strategies 177
 Physical Health Strategies 178
 Organizational Strategies 179

LEGAL & DISCLAIMER

The information contained in this book is not designed to replace or take the place of any form of medicine or professional medical advice. The information in this book has been provided for educational and entertainment purposes only.

The information contained in this book has been compiled from sources deemed reliable, and it is accurate to the best of the Author's knowledge; however, the Author cannot guarantee its accuracy and validity and cannot be held liable for any errors or omissions. Changes are periodically made to this book. You must consult your doctor or get professional medical advice before using any of the suggested remedies, techniques, or information in this book.

Upon using the information contained in this book, you agree to hold harmless the Author from and against any damages, costs, and expenses, including any legal fees potentially resulting from the application of any of the information provided by this guide. This disclaimer applies to any damages or injury caused by the use and application, whether directly or indirectly, of any advice or information presented, whether for breach of contract, tort, negligence, personal injury, criminal intent, or under any other cause of action.

You agree to accept all risks of using the information presented inside this book. You need to consult a professional medical practitioner in order to ensure you are both able and healthy enough to participate in this program

FREE BONUS REPORT

https://mailchi.mp/984c5b627dda/freebonusresource

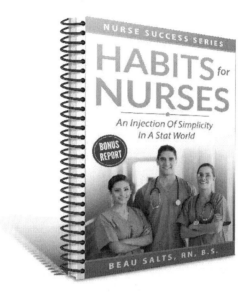

Join my email list to receive future book release alerts. You will also receive this free bonus report, which includes:

> ➢ *Hacks for spending less time doing house chores!*
> ➢ *Triple your storage space!*
> ➢ *Specific product recommendations to make your life easier!*

Get your **free** bonus report at:

https://mailchi.mp/984c5b627dda/freebonusresource

INTRODUCTION

Are you a nurse who is feeling overwhelmed by the stresses of the job, the long hours, and the requests to work extra shifts? Do you feel that the profession is sometimes so demanding that it saps your energy, robs you of your free time, and directly contributes to your lack of a personal life? I know I do.

This book has been a labor of love, and I am thrilled that it has finally found its way into your hands. It is all about nurses and upping our quality of life. We are busy people. Not only on the job, but in our personal lives as well. Many of us work long shifts. Some of us work long shifts PLUS have a long commute to work.

When I worked medical-surgical, my shift was twelve hours, plus I had an hour commute to and from work. Many other nurses are in similar situations, and our home lives are strained because of the long work hours. This book is all about making simple and practical self-improvements.

Allow me to introduce myself. I am Beau Salts, and I work full-time as a registered nurse. I also happen to have a thing for dumping the contents of my brain onto paper in a form that is useful to others.

As a male nurse, I have been mistaken countless times for a "doctor" or a "pharmacist." I have had patients instinctively answer a question I asked, "yes ma'am, er, I mean yes sir." Does it bother me? Not one bit. Remember this—what matters is what you think of yourself, not what others think of you. What other people think of you is none of your business.

I have worked medical-surgical, outpatient hemodialysis, and psychiatric. Everyone knows med-surg is hectic, but I would say outpatient HD was a level above med-surg in the "insanely fast-paced and stressful" department. HD was unbelievably busy.

It was either sink or swim, and I learned so many lessons there. My time-management skills were honed, and I learned to operate in an environment that would make many people have a meltdown. Anyone that has worked a few "changeovers" knows exactly what I am talking about.

I have lived and learned, and I continue to look

forward to learning new life lessons every day. I am sure that you could share many lessons with me as well and I would love to hear what you have to say. I believe that as nurses, we should all be in this together.

In my experience, most nurses are very helpful with one another. There are exceptions, just as there are in any line of work or endeavor. But the majority are willing to help each other. As a case-in-point, when I worked medical-surgical, there were times when I would give another nurse's patient a pain medication, so that nurse's lunch break would not have to be disturbed. Other nurses would often help me in this manner and many other ways.

More experienced nurses can help newer nurses as the newbies encounter inevitable situations that school somehow didn't fully prepare them for. I believe that when we help one another, the entire profession benefits.

Not only that, our patients and their families also benefit. When nurses help other nurses, what we essentially have is a giant "think tank" where all of our individual knowledge and experiences collide. I would argue that two brains are better than one, and three brains are better than two.

While the book does not contain solutions to every problem we may face, it does provide new ways of thinking about common problems and unique ways of attacking the challenges that we face. My intention is that the angles I present will help make our lives easier, more organized, efficient, and enjoyable.

I am far from perfect, but I have been in the trenches, made mistakes, and learned from them. I am now passing these lessons on, and I trust that they will touch lives.

This book is the inaugural edition of a series of books on success habits for nurses. The series will take a holistic approach to success in nursing, including tactics to help both on the job and at home, because it is all connected.

Topics that we will dive into include self-improvement (both personally and professionally), making exercise practical (and getting it DONE), user-friendly nutrition, communications, back health, putting chores on autopilot, and more.

This first book will serve as the kick-off and will explore a variety of topics that are infinitely relevant to a nurse's life. This book will go into some level of depth on each topic but will not be totally comprehensive. Topics will be dissected further in upcoming books, and new fresh topics will be covered as well.

Perhaps you are busy helping your kids with their homework every night or taking care of your four dogs. Whatever the case may be, our goal is to free up time in as many areas of our life as possible. The overall effect will be a net gain of free time, or at the very least, less feeling overwhelmed and more confidence that we "have it together."

As the title suggests, I am here to help my fellow nurses simplify their lives. I am an enormous believer in the power of simplicity. You won't find any complicated solutions here. When was the last time a complicated solution actually worked for you? (I am hearing crickets now.) They don't work for me, either. We don't have time for that. What you WILL find are workable solutions to real-world problems that confront nurses on a daily basis.

At the time of this writing, all the links that are included in this book are active and functional. Should you notice that a link is not working, please email me, and I will correct the issue. You can contact me at:

admin@beausalts.com

MENTAL STRATEGIES

RITUALS

Rituals are invaluable in our lives because they become positive habits that we eventually repeat without even thinking about it. I recommend having a ritual for morning, mid-day, and bedtime. I am going to give some examples of solid rituals, but feel free to incorporate your own personalized ideas as well.

When you're a nurse, you are forced to deal with a lot of uncertainty and surprises. It's just the nature of your work. There's a myriad of possibilities that could take place in any typical workday. A stable patient might seemingly develop complications out of nowhere, and you would have to address it. A natural disaster might take place nearby, inflicting damage on dozens of people, and your hospital has to care for an influx of patients. You just never really know what kind of stress is in store for you on any given workday. All of that uncertainty can only add to the stress of your job. It might feel like too many things are happening which are beyond your control, and that's not a good feeling to have over an extended period. It could potentially drive you to having constant anxiety and fear in your profession.

This is why it's very important for you to add a sense of structure and purpose to your everyday life in the form of habits and routines. This way, not all aspects of your life are seemingly beyond your control. When you make an effort to practice healthy routines, you are taking more control over your life. And this is going to help do wonders for your mental health and psyche. On top of that, having a solid routine for you to fall back on will help you be more efficient with the way you conduct your work. If you need some ideas, here is a sample routine that you can use on a typical workday.

MORNING ROUTINE:

- As soon as your feet hit the floor, do one minute of exercise to get yourself ready to conquer the day. This can be a minute of a cardio exercise such as "fast feet" or "jumping jacks."

- Have a drink of your filtered water to re-hydrate when you get out of bed.
- As you go about getting ready for the day, be aware of your thoughts. Purposely focus on everything you are grateful for. Also, make it a point to feed your mind with positive thoughts by telling yourself at least five positive messages.
- Also, think about what you want to accomplish with this new day you have been blessed with, and visualize the day as a huge success.

MID-DAY ROUTINE:

- You need to "de-stress" in the middle of your day. There is a good chance that you have encountered some stressors in your day up until this point, and you need to nuke them and get them off your plate. Go somewhere private for one to two minutes and get it all out of your head and into your journal, whether that is written or audio. If you have a trusted confidante at work that you can share things with, that will work also.
- During your one- to two-minute "mid-day jolt," also do something physical while you are in a private area. This will further help

rid your body of stress hormones and bring some endorphins on-board. Thirty seconds of jumping jacks or jogging in place are good options.
- If you do caffeine, this might be a good time to partake of it. It can help give you a little extra "push" to get you ready to conquer the second half of the day.

NIGHT-TIME ROUTINE:

- One excellent way to relax your body and mind in preparation for sleep is to take a warm bath. Adding Epsom salts to the bathwater will further help relax you because it contains magnesium, which has a calming effect. You can also add calming essential oils such as lavender.
- Having an essential oil diffuser by your bed is a good idea. There are many essential oils available, and you can pick them based on your goal. For example, to help with sleep, lavender is an excellent choice.
- Before bed, we want to purge the day and clear our minds. One good way to do this is to do five minutes of journaling before bed. You can either write or record your thoughts on audio, whichever you prefer.

Journal anything and everything that is bothering you, good things that happened today, lessons, whatever. Just get it out of your head so that your mind can be at peace, and you can enter a restful slumber.
- In the last thirty minutes or so that you are preparing for bed, I recommend the use of blue light glasses. These will dramatically limit the amount of light entering the retinas of your eyes and will help to increase melatonin production. This, in turn, will promote sleepiness. You will find an excellent option for these glasses in the appendix.
- Peaceful sounds can help promote relaxation and sleep, and can "drown out" any undesired sounds that may disturb you. Some options for this include a white noise machine or a smartphone app such as the Sleep Sounds app. If you prefer music over other sounds, the musician Enya is an excellent choice for calming music.
- As you lay down in bed, this is the ideal time to meditate. Consult the meditation section in this book for a simple meditation technique that will bring your attention to your breathing and help to clear your mind, both of which will promote sleep.

Of course, these are just examples of things that you can do to add a sense of structure to your life. Ultimately, it's up to you on what kind of habits you would want to enforce on yourself. Ideally, the routines that you engage in would be ones that might actually add a lot of value to your life. Read books or listen to good music. Exercise and stay healthy. Meditate and engage in self-reflection. These are just some great examples of ways in which you can be more structured with your day while also doing things that are meaningful and fulfilling.

SELF-IMPROVEMENT 2020

There is a multitude of self-help books out there, many of which I had read when I was pursuing my psychology degree. Of all of them that I have read, there are a few principles that stand out. Principles that really work and are infinitely applicable to our lives. One such principle is to do the work first, THEN reward yourself. Not the reverse.

Let's say you have a day off, and you have a goal or goals you want to get done. You also have something fun you want to do, something you really look forward to doing. Maybe you have been meaning to watch a certain movie for weeks, but you have been too busy up until now, and you finally have the opportunity.

It will be in your best interest to pour your energy into accomplishing the goals first, then watch the movie as a reward. The movie will also provide something to look forward to while you are working on the goal.

In making changes in our lives, it is crucial to do your most important tasks early in the day. Why do it this way? The main reason is we have limited energy each day. We need to be sure we have the energy for the most important things by doing them first.

When you wake up in the morning, jump out of bed with passion and excitement for the new day, the new beginning that you have been blessed with. Immediately, start telling yourself positive messages. Get started immediately on constructive activities. You should already have a loose plan and a general idea of what you want to accomplish for the day. You should also prioritize the things you want and need to get done.

You should always strive to balance work and play. And you can even bring some play to your work. How, you might ask? An example would be finding the humor in daily affairs at work. Perhaps you and your coworkers can laugh some sticky situations off instead of taking them seriously and stressing yourself out. Get the idea? Good.

We only have a limited amount of energy, or lifeblood as I like to call it, available each day. You can choose to spend your lifeblood in meaningful, constructive pursuits, or you can choose to waste it with meaningless pursuits. Again, I believe in balance. But it is crucial to refrain from the play until the work is done.

The play can serve as a reward, something to look forward to after the work is done. And if you should fail to get the work done, you must punish yourself by refraining from the play. This is much the same as a parent may deal with his or her child, and it is a very effective system. If you do what you're supposed to do, you get the carrot. If you don't, you get the stick. Simple, time-tested, and effective.

MOMENTUM

There are three words in particular that I believe will have the most impact on your self-improvement efforts. Those three words are MO MEN TUM. This is where it's at folks. The thing is, momentum can work for us or against us.

As a personal example, I once got into a kick where I would come home from work, lay down on the couch before doing anything, and stay there for HOURS. I would lay there from like 7:30 in the evening to around 1:00 AM when I should have been spending that prime time wisely.

I just started doing this a time or two, and soon it became an ongoing pattern that I found very difficult to break out of. When I would finally drag myself off the couch in the wee hours of the morning, I would realize that I had not yet had dinner, and I would go have "dinner" at this crazy hour.

Many other basic self-care activities were being neglected as well, to say nothing of all the goals I had that were going untouched. Being stuck in this rut made me feel terrible about myself.

Neglecting ourselves like this DOES have a negative impact on our self-esteem, our motivation and productivity, and our mental and physical health. This goes to show how easy it is for us to slide into ridiculously bad habits, basically just because we repeated it and got used to the pattern.

Once our body's "habit Cadillac" gets stuck on "park," it is not easy to shift it into "drive." Sorry, I couldn't resist the metaphor. ☺ No, it's not easy by any means. But it is SIMPLE. The key is shifting the momentum in the direction we know we need to go.

Another principle from self-improvement I have

observed time and time again to be true is that when we want change in our lives, we must act FAST. To delay, to procrastinate, is to sign our own contract for failure. When we feel the need for change, action is the only thing that will bring about that change. And action will kick-start your momentum.

MOMENTUM — TAKE ACTION

Use momentum to your advantage. Take some positive action NOW. It does not matter how seemingly small that action is. Any action will get you moving in the right direction. If you've been meaning to start exercising but haven't done so in months, DO SOMETHING. Maybe you aren't 100% gung-ho yet about committing to working out, but you know you should, and part of you really wants to. If you can't yet bring yourself to do an entire workout, just do a fraction of a workout. To get the momentum working in your favor, just do one set of an exercise. Even small bits of effort like this will help get the momentum going and help you bust out of the prison of your comfort zone.

Continue doing fractions of workouts as the days go along, gradually increasing what you do until you start doing full workouts. Note that this advice is only intended for those of you who tend to procrastinate on the regular and avoid working out. If you are already motivated and able to do full workouts, that is fantastic. Just be aware of the principle of momentum. Basically, whatever we do (or don't do) tends to get repeated. Hence, the term habit. Be proactive and ensure that momentum works for you and helps move you toward your goals.

INFLUENCES

Do not think for a second that your day-to-day actions have no bearing on your self-esteem, overall mental health, and future. I have found that day-to-day activities have everything to do with our futures. The choices we make today profoundly affect our tomorrows. And I don't just mean the big choices. I mean every choice.

Think about it this way. What type of life am I setting myself up for if I stay up to ridiculously late hours every night watching movies and tv shows, and sleep late every morning, finally dragging out of bed when the better part of the day has already passed? Not a very good one. You see, by the actions I choose to engage in, and by the actions I choose to refrain from today, I am choosing how my tomorrow will go.

Everything we allow into our minds will have an

effect on us, positive or negative. Every little thing we are exposed to has some influence on us. It is imperative that we start putting more thought into what influences we allow into our lives.

We must really question the television, movies, music, games, other people, etc. that we choose to take part in. These things truly have a profound impact on our lives. Perhaps you are like I was in the past. I did not believe these things had much of an effect on me and so I just brushed it off as unimportant. But I have come to realize that yes, these things DO make a difference, and they ARE important. Let me explain it this way.

Even if we are not consciously aware of the negative influences, they are running in the background in our subconscious mind. As the old axiom goes, garbage in, garbage out. Let's pay close attention to the things we allow to influence us. We must guard our minds, just as a security guard protects and guards his post.

CONTROL YOUR THOUGHTS

There is something almost addictive about continuing in our loop of negative thinking. In my own experience, I have found this to be true. There is also the mindset of, "well, I have gone this far down this wrong road, so what is the use in turning around now?" But let me urge you to resist that type of thinking. I don't care if you have gone 500 miles in the wrong direction. TURN AROUND. Get moving in the right direction!

Here is the best method I have found for controlling our thoughts. First of all, we have to be on guard constantly. In the beginning, we will have to consciously remind ourselves, but soon the habit will set in, and this will be automatic. Awareness is the key. When a thought crosses your mind that you believe is a negative message, use your mind's eye to destroy it. Remember the giant rolling stone that almost flattened Indiana Jones? (For the younger crowd—if you don't get this movie reference, Google it already ☺). Imagine that enormous, mind-bogglingly heavy stone being dropped from an airplane and landing on your negative thought. Feel the earth shake violently under your feet, and hear the earth-shattering sound of the massive rock colliding with the earth. Now notice that the negative thought that was just harassing you has "left the building." The thought was totally obliterated, and now you have a clean slate to work with. Start filling your mind with positive messages now, whatever those are for you.

We have to be aware of what we are thinking. Would you allow someone else to talk to you that way? And here you are talking to yourself far worse than you would allow another person to talk to you.

Remember, the thoughts you think are like sentences and words being spoken to you out loud by someone else. The mind does register the thoughts you think and responds to them accordingly. You have to always remember this and take your thoughts seriously.

We must control our thoughts. It is ultimately the actions we take or do not take that will change our lives, but the thoughts we think will determine those actions. The source of change is the mind. But the engine that births that change is ACTION.

Ultimately, it is our actions that are of supreme importance. Our actions feed back into our thoughts and influence subsequent thoughts, which influence subsequent actions. It is something of a cycle. What input goes into the cycle determines what product comes out. We must be guardians of our minds and consciously choose the input that goes in.

Remember, the activities we engage in, the actions we take or do not take, all send messages to our subconscious minds. This, in turn, affects our self-esteem for the better or worse, depending on the things we do or don't do. It is our deeds that determine our destinies. And yes, our deeds originate in our thoughts, so the old axiom "we become what we think about" that was popularized by Earl Nightingale in the 1950s does hold true so long as our actions are in line with our thoughts.

The importance of delayed gratification, sacrifice, and engaging in meaningful, wholesome activities cannot be overstated. We must purge the meaningless, wasteful activities from our lives without compromise. We must be ruthless in this regard.

To be clear, I am absolutely not saying we shouldn't have fun. Having fun is an enormously important part of staying happy and healthy. Just be thoughtful about what you choose for entertainment and the message it will send to your subconscious.

ADDICTION

Are you struggling with some type of personal demon that you would like to bid farewell, but you just can't seem to shake it? If so, your demon may actually be a full-fledged addiction. If you have something like this in your life that you truly want to part ways with, a holistic approach is best.

Combining every available effective method and resource that you have at your disposal is the best approach. We cannot beat a powerful addiction with a casual, half-hearted effort. We have to wage an all-out war.

I am going to provide one weapon for the war, but again, you need an entire arsenal. I encourage you to explore further and utilize everything available to you, whether that be professional therapies, medication, or the many other options out there. Again, addiction eradication is best approached in a holistic manner. If you are interested, I can delve deeper into this in a future book.

The first step is to formally commit to beating the addiction. Writing down your commitment is a vital part. If you want to keep it private, nobody has to see this but you.

A key principle in the war against addiction is to remember that there have to be consequences for our actions. Consequences are motivating to us. Consequences get us moving and taking action. Consequences make things happen or halt certain actions in their tracks.

If you know for a fact that if you throw trash out the window of your car, that a cop is going to hunt you down and write you a ticket and force you to pay a $10,000 fine, my guess is that you would be very motivated not to throw your trash out the window.

Examples of this can go on and on, but you get the message. If we are struggling with a particular area of our lives where we are trying to change but failing over and over again, consider this: IN ORDER TO ELIMINATE AN ADDICTION, THERE MUST BE REAL CONSEQUENCES FOR NOT ELIMINATING THE ADDICTION. In practical terms, when I am feeling the urge to engage in the addiction, there must be an IMMEDIATE negative consequence if I give in and indulge the addiction.

The common knowledge seems to be that addiction is too powerful to be beaten with rational thought. That to truly motivate ourselves, we must work with our emotions instead of our logical minds. In my experience, this is not entirely the case. I have noticed that when it comes down to it, we usually have a conversation with ourselves before we do or do not do something.

For instance, I feel an urge to engage in my addiction one day. When I start feeling the urge, a conversation starts in my head. I am telling myself the reasons I want to oblige the urge and the reasons I shouldn't. Ok, that is the moment it all comes down to. The defining moment.

It is my belief that our logical minds have more power than they have been given credit for in these situations. At this critical moment, I CAN tell myself, "NO. I will not feed this addiction." And instead of giving in to the urge, I can go do something else. It truly is that simple. Simplicity is beautiful. Curing our addictions need not be complicated. What we need are strategies we will actually USE. Simple strategies fit that bill like nothing else.

In many cases, we only change when we have to. We do things out of necessity. This is the true motivator, the thing that will get us moving and taking action when nothing else will. To try to change by other means will almost certainly result in procrastination, laziness, quitting, and ultimately failure.

We have to put ourselves in situations where we MUST change. Where we face serious consequences for not changing. This is the only way—the way to true change.

I do believe the pleasure/pain psychology is useful and very necessary to leverage. However, we CAN motivate ourselves by simply deciding to say yay or nay in that critical moment. It all comes down to that moment when we are waging war with the urge. All of this discussion comes down to that. These are the moments that determine our destinies. And you determine how these moments will play out.

After you have made your decision, your entire day will go down a different path depending on what you chose. And the way this day goes will drastically influence how tomorrow goes. Such is the makeup of our lives.

HOW TO FIGHT BACK

I am now going to roll out a powerful tactic for fighting addiction. Think of some things you dislike. We are going to harness the power of these negative associations to not only overcome our addictions, but to laugh in their face.

As an example, let's say I am a smoker, and I want to toss this addiction. Yes, it is totally possible to simply decide to quit and to do so. However, the odds are not in our favor if we use that approach alone. Most of us simply do not have that degree of willpower. Actually, we do have it deep inside; we simply are not in touch with it.

We need an approach that will help make our aspirations of being free from the addiction a reality. I am going to accept the impulse as it floods over me. I am going to be honest with myself that yes, I am indeed vulnerable at this moment in time to giving in to this powerful force known as an addiction.

I can't stand mustard. If I order a hamburger without it yet find when I get home from the drive-thru that it was put on anyway, I will actually scrape it off. I may even throw away the hamburger altogether. I dislike mustard THAT much. Having said that, I can use this to my advantage when it comes to slaying an addiction, and so can you.

Continuing with our smoking example—let's say I am trying to kick the habit. I have already made a formal commitment to myself, including writing it down. Now I need to have specific, effective tactics planned out in advance. If I don't, I am setting myself up for failure. Realistically, this is going to be hard. It may even seem impossible at times.

Knowing that, I need to go into this battle armed with ways of fighting back. This will help catapult me over and beyond the moments of truth, as I call them. These are the moments in time that it all comes down to.

Our choices in these defining moments will determine how our immediate futures and our long-term destinies play out. Sounds like a lot of pressure, doesn't it? Not to worry, with this system, we will be prepared to come out with the victory.

We have to revisit that word—consequences. In this particular example, I am going to take advantage of the fact that I find mustard to be repulsive. I am going to carry around a small packet of mustard in my pocket, where it will lie in wait for the next time I am waging war with my addiction.

When an impulse to smoke comes, as it inevitably will, I am not going to attempt to ignore the impulse. After all, most of us have been trying the brute strength approach to quitting over and over, to no avail. It's time for a different approach.

This is where the mustard packet comes in to play. I have to tell myself that if I give in to this urge, I am going to have to face the immediate consequence of eating this entire packet of mustard. I have to be 100% committed to following through on that consequence.

When my mind starts considering this new scenario, with the element of consequence thrown into the mix, it now has reason to really pause and think about this whole thing. My brain perks up and pays attention to the reality in front of it. A side benefit is that thinking about both the cigarettes and the mustard simultaneously can actually help the existing negative association to the mustard carry over to the cigarettes.

Once I present my brain with this scenario, now there is a real deterrent to firing up. I now know that if I do it, I am seriously going to have to eat an entire packet of this delicacy that I detest. Human psychology dictates that we will do more to avoid pain than to gain pleasure.

Now that I have an option in front of me to either receive the guaranteed immediate pleasure of smoking or the immediate guaranteed pain of the consequence, I am going to choose to avoid the pain. What happens if I somehow manage to choose the habit I am trying to break?

In that case, as soon as I am done with that cigarette, I have a tasty packet of mustard waiting for me that I am going to have to grin and bear. A time or two of that, and I am going to really start rethinking this whole cigarette thing.

The key to this method is that you have to be committed to following through on your consequence if you choose to indulge your addiction. In other words, if you give in to the addiction, you WILL initiate your chosen consequence.

Pick something that is personalized to you and your sensibilities. Also, be sure it is practical. For instance, if you choose taking a cold tub bath as your consequence, that will only be viable if you are at home at the time of engagement in the addiction. Depending on what you are struggling with, you may need an option that you can use wherever you are.

This is something that you need to come up with yourself. Be honest with yourself. What is something that will really work for YOU? What do you have an existing STRONG negative association to that will truly deter you? Is it practical for your addiction? Can it be immediately implemented?

Some examples:

A. cold bath
B. if you dislike mayonnaise or ketchup, this is a good option due to the portability of the packets
C. if you are shy, make yourself do something embarrassing that will call a lot of attention to you (obviously this one would only work in public)
D. the possibilities are only limited by your imagination

These would deter me, but they may not deter every reader. If they do deter you, then great, feel free to use these. Again, this is something you will have to personalize.

This is a way to get some serious leverage on ourselves. The notion that we have to "hit rock bottom" in order to change has some truth to it. One way or another, we have to "wake up," see reality, and feel the need to change. More often than not, it is going to be pain that drives us to change.

This method is not "nice" or even "politically correct." It is a bit unorthodox. But it will work for you if you work it.

I believe we are all capable of holding ourselves accountable to the consequence. However, if you insist that you can't, you will need to leverage an accountability partner. Give this partner permission to make you implement the consequence should you fail to make yourself. If necessary, have an agreement that you can call or text your partner at any time the need arises.

I am not here to sell you on the idea of quitting smoking, or any other addiction for that matter. We are nurses, and we are smart people. We have already heard the reasons a million times. It comes down to this...do YOU want to quit? The decision to continue an addiction or not is yours. However, if you choose to quit, that is where these methods can help you bring that notion to fruition.

I have had countless patients in the hospital and psychiatric setting that were smokers, some heavy smokers. I can tell you from experience with hundreds of patients that the nicotine patch DOES WORK. If smoking is the addiction you are fighting, use it as part of your plan of attack.

Another facet of this strategy is to think of all the logical reasons you have for wanting to make this change in your life. What are your reasons for seeking to destroy this addiction? Get very clear on these reasons and document them on paper, audio, or any medium that works best for you.

Of course, we should utilize other established and proven methods in conjunction with these psychological strategies. Remember, a holistic approach to health, wellness, and most everything related to this is best.

The pain/pleasure psychology has been around for ages. I am not contributing anything new or groundbreaking here in terms of principles. Where many other resources fall short, however, is in translating these ivory tower theories into the HERE and NOW of our lives. Sometimes they leave us feeling high and dry. What I am doing here is filling in the gap between sound psychological principle and relevance to our lives.

The actions we take tend to get repeated. The thoughts we think tend to get repeated. And the more we reinforce our actions or thoughts, the more they become ingrained in our psyche and our physicality, and the more they become "us." To apply this knowledge to addiction, the more we resist our addiction, the easier it will be to resist it the next time we are confronted with an urge.

KEEP CALM

As nurses, being able to maintain a peaceful interior and a professional exterior are essential. Doing this is much easier said than done, though, wouldn't you agree? Just talking about this and dreaming or hoping that we can make it happen is not enough. We need strategies. Unless you happen to have the patience of Job or the inner peace of the Dalai Lama, this is something you are going to have to work at.

You know as well as I do that nursing can be incredibly hectic at times. Even the majority of the time. It seems like one million tasks are thrown at you at once, and you have to scratch and claw just to keep your head above water.

Maybe your nurse manager calls for a huddle just when you were about to start that IV you had been trying to get to all day. Or maybe a patient's family member stops you in the hall for updates when all you want to do is finish your charting to get home on time. Or your clock-watching patient requests his q2h prn IV hydromorphone 5 minutes early when you were about to hang a new bag of TPN. And one of my personal pet peeves is having to hunt down medications that pharmacy has not stocked in the medication machine. Having to stop what I am doing and getting out of my "groove" to go look for a medication is infinitely irritating. Can anyone relate?

Yes, to say that interruptions and frustrations abound would be an understatement. There truly is a constant flow of do this, do that. I have found that it is just the nature of the profession, especially in areas like medical-surgical. But as one of my former bosses always said, "if you can't handle the heat, get out of the kitchen." We have committed to this profession.

Therefore, it does us no good to whine and complain (unless we are whining and complaining while also doing something about it). Yes, it is good to vent your frustrations to a confidante. We do have to have outlets for our stresses.

But please don't be the one that is constantly griping, complaining, and finding fault. Such is the nurse that no one wants to be around, and quite frankly, contributes to a toxic environment. There is a stark difference in being a chronic complainer, and a person that expresses his or her displeasure in a productive manner. To be productive, we have to stay positive and look for solutions.

Having said that, we are medical professionals. Patients aren't supposed to see us sweat. We have to keep our composure, at least in front of patients and colleagues. We have to maintain our professional image. After all, if we don't have it together, how can patients look to us for guidance? What we need are simple, actionable techniques that can help us keep our calm on.

Before nursing, I studied psychology at a university, which culminated in a bachelor of science degree. I learned so much about stress, anxiety, worry, depression; you name it. I have also been a voracious reader of all topics psychology-related.

Other nurses have often commented on my ability to remain calm, even when it seems that bombs and rockets and hurricanes of demands and tasks are exploding and roaring all around. It is all about your psychology. For the first time, I am going to disclose some awesome tactics that will help you maintain your serenity.

MEET MAXIMUS

Do you happen to have a 400-pound pet gorilla? Yeah, me neither—it would cost way too much to feed him. However, that doesn't mean that we can't IMAGINE a 400-pound gorilla. And in so doing, we can release some of our negative energy and stress. How? Read on.

I am going to unveil one of my unique spins on visualization, with the goal of helping other nurses to keep it together mentally and emotionally. And for that matter, to THRIVE mentally and emotionally and be STRONG.

Remember, we are role models for our patients and colleagues. This technique is meant to be used in real-time, when you are feeling frustrated, stressed, or just feeling negative energy for whatever reason.

Again, things happen in this profession pretty much constantly that can invoke these types of feelings. It is important that we RELEASE the negative energy. Carrying it around is simply not healthy, and I would argue that doing so will not only lead to job dissatisfaction and underperformance but will also bleed over into your personal life. It's all connected. Not to mention, harboring this type of negativity perpetually is a really good way to wind up in an early grave.

Getting back to our pet 400-pound gorilla, and how he relates to crushing our negative feelings, whether these are frustration, anger, worry, disappointment, heartbreak, fear, or any other. What you want to do is imagine a big, strong, heavy gorilla. You can name him or her if you want, and even put the beast on a leash if it floats your boat.

In any event, what you do is think of this gorilla when you are hit with these negative feelings that stress you out, in real-time as you are having the feelings. Let's say you are an hour behind on your morning medication pass, struggling to get caught up, and you hear you are getting a new admission in twenty minutes. This is enough to stress the best of us out to the max and beyond.

This is where our pet gorilla can help. As an example, I will call my gorilla Maximus, and I just found myself in the scenario of already being behind and learning that I am getting an admission thrown into the mix. Nurses know that admissions are one of the most time-consuming and work-intensive parts of the job.

Panicking is not going to help here. What will help is maintaining our inner, focused calm. We need to accept the negative energy that this situation provokes. We need to take three to five SLOW, deep breaths, while at the same time beginning our visualization.

The slow deep breaths are key because they trigger the parasympathetic nervous system, which helps to slow things down, such as your heart rate. When I say slow, you want to take a good seven seconds for your inhalation, hold your breath for seven seconds, and then exhale slowly for seven seconds. Do not rush it. Take the full seven seconds. If you rush it, you will defeat the purpose of the exercise. Slow breaths will help our heart rate slow down

MENTAL STRATEGIES

and will help our racing mind to come back within the speed limit.

In your mind, take the negative energy, and vacuum it up into a small black box, similar to how the Ghostbusters vacuum up ghosts into their ghost trap. Once the problem and its associated negative energy are trapped inside the box, toss the box onto the floor.

Now order Maximus to STOMP IT. Upon your command, imagine that your 400-pound gorilla jumps up and down, up and down on top of the small black box. Maximus bounces on it repeatedly, and each time he lands, you can feel the earth shake violently.

You can feel the vibrations starting in your feet and moving all the way up your body, making their exit through the top of your head. Take three to five more SLOW deep breaths.

Maximus continues to jump up and down and totally CRUSH the black box, which contains your problem and negative energy, into oblivion. There is nothing but a cloud of fine dust left when he stops. A strong draft comes along and sweeps the dust away into nothingness.

As the energy is swept away, feel a powerful peace flood your body and mind. Think of something you love, whether that be coming home to your dog, a favorite memory, or a favorite place. Anything that will help flood your mind and body with positivity.

After Maximus has crushed our demons, we don't just have a lack of negativity now. We also have a new surge of positive energy, strength, and determination to succeed. Take a moment to really FEEL these empowering emotions. Feel a rush of overwhelming determination, as if nothing can stop you, and you can not only handle whatever you face, but you can actually laugh in these problems' face, so to speak. Now bask in the inner peace. You are now ok with this situation. You are a nurse, an astute professional, and deep inside a fighter, and you are ready to handle this.

And just like that, the negative energy that your problem triggered has been CRUSHED. This entire process will take you less than a minute, and you can repeat it as many 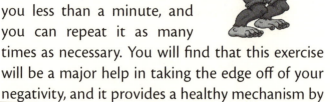 times as necessary. You will find that this exercise will be a major help in taking the edge off of your negativity, and it provides a healthy mechanism by which you can RELEASE the energy.

Visualization is nothing new. It has been proven time and time again. The problem is, figuring out practical ways to implement it into our everyday lives has been a challenge. Now you have a simple, fun technique that shows you exactly how to harness the power of visualization.

SQUEEZE

Another option for releasing negative energy is to squeeze something in your hand. Working out helps tremendously with getting rid of the bad energy, but it is not practical at all times in the work setting. Therefore, find something to keep in your scrubs pocket that you can take out and squeeze when needed. You can even squeeze it while it's still in your pocket if you need to be discreet.

Whatever item works for you and is practical and portable. Whether it is a small rubber ball or a commercial product like "Therapy Putty," find what works for you. Squeezing this item in your hand when all heck breaks loose serves as a release mechanism and will help you stay on track.

SLEEP

Everyone needs sleep. This is the only time of the day when you literally get to shut your body down and recuperate. As a nurse, you're working very long hours during your shifts. And it's not like you have the kind of job where you're just sitting around doing mindless work either (not that there's anything wrong with that). Being the amazing nursing professional that you are, you're always on your feet. You're always up and about. You have to constantly monitor different patients and keep yourself updated with all sorts of different cases.

There's no denying that this kind of profession is particularly straining, not just on the body, but also on the mind. One of the best ways to address whatever exhaustion or fatigue you're feeling is getting enough sleep at night. And we're not just talking about the quantity here. You need to get QUALITY sleep too. You might already be familiar with sleep cycles. But to brush you up on it, sleep stages are composed of four levels:

A. Awake
B. REM (Rapid Eye Movement)
C. Light Sleep
D. Deep Sleep

Your goal every night is to get as much deep sleep as possible. This is where your mind and your body really shut down and recover. Amazing things happen to your body when you get quality sleep. If you're having trouble getting quality sleep at night, here are a few things you can do:

MEDITATE BEFORE SLEEPING

Meditation is one of the best ways to get you to fall asleep. Usually, your body will start to feel relaxed and sleepy when you lower your heart rate. One of the most effective ways of lowering your heart rate is by practicing mindful breathing through meditation. Even just a 5-minute meditation session can really help you fall asleep easier.

DIFFUSE LAVENDER ESSENTIAL OILS

There are all sorts of essential oils out there that can help induce drowsiness and relaxation. However, lavender essential oil seems to be the one that people respond most effectively to. It is an essential oil that has some soothing and relaxing properties that can help condition your mind for sleep.

TURN DOWN THE TEMPERATURE IN YOUR BEDROOM

Studies have shown that people tend to fall asleep easier whenever the temperature of the room that they are in falls on the cooler side of the spectrum (Doheny, 2008). In fact, not only do people fall asleep more easily, they also tend to get better quality sleep under cooler conditions.

SLEEP IN A COMPLETELY DARK ROOM

This will assist your body in producing melatonin. To help you accomplish this, blackout curtains are ideal. Check out the appendix for a quality blackout curtain option.

EMOTIONAL STRATEGIES

COMMUNICATIONS

When you're a nurse, you have to understand the importance of communication. Being an effective communicator makes all the difference in the workplace—with both your patients and your coworkers.

If you fail to communicate well, then you put yourself at a distinct disadvantage. Everyone wants to succeed but to succeed, you need the right tools, and that's exactly what I will provide to you.

BEDSIDE MANNER

There is nothing more valuable to you as a nurse than having a good bedside manner. Yes, your years of medical experience are important as well, but that means naught if you have no way to communicate with your patients properly.

Your bedside manner is the determining factor in what type of relationship you will foster with your patient. We treat people how we want them to treat us. One thing I always tell other people is to imagine being the one in the hospital bed or chair. How would you want to be spoken to and treated?

Of course, you might already know that bedside manner is important. After all, the nursing school you went to probably drilled it into your mind that you should be respectful and kind to all patients. However, there is a difference between what you're told at school and actually practicing your bedside manner with patients.

I get it. It's hard when you have your own personal problems weighing on your shoulders. Perhaps you didn't get enough sleep last night, or you messed up, and your supervisor chewed you out. It's easy to revert into our own personal spaces when we aren't feeling 100%. This makes relating to our patients a little harder.

Your bedside manner should be practiced every day and with every patient. Your patients are vulnerable, and many might be scared of what they are in the hospital for. Medical terminology might go over their heads, and you are their safety net.

When your bedside manner envelopes them with understanding and respect, you help assuage those fears and make your patient more comfortable. I know this can be hard to remember as you move from patient to patient, so take a few tips that will help you improve your bedside manner.

- Don't be stingy with that smile of yours. A smile is your first step toward showing your patient that you have a welcoming attitude. Enter every room with a smile so that your patients don't feel like they are unwanted or a burden. When you allow your negativity to bleed into your facial features, your patient's demeanor will suffer as well. Be mindful that there are times when you are handling patients and delicate information where smiling might not be appropriate; however, you still want to give off as much positive energy as possible.
- Be focused on your patient. The minute you walk into the walls of your work, your personal issues need to remain at the door. You can't properly help your patient if your mind is stuck on the issues in your home. Your goal should be to give your patients the best care you can that focuses on them and their health.
- Always show your patient respect. Many nurses become confused at this point. How do you demonstrate your respect for your patients? Well, you can begin by

understanding and researching the different cultural backgrounds of your patients. As a nurse, you will meet people from all walks of life. When you encounter someone new from a culture you have no experience with, it doesn't hurt to do a little bit of research to make sure you're respecting them and their beliefs. This will cement a foundation with your patients. If you make promises to a patient, follow through. If a patient requests to speak to other team members, allow them to do so. Honoring the patient's needs to the best of your ability is a great way to show respect.

- Don't half-listen to your patient. Active listening is an essential part of having a good bedside manner. This means that you provide your patient with all of your concentration by showing that you are interested and listening through your facial expressions, body language, and verbalizing what they are requesting. Active listening is the best tool in your arsenal because it truly allows you to be your patient's best advocate.
- Finally, don't be shy about asking your patient questions. Always ask your patient how you can best help them and make sure that you offer final help to them before

moving on to your next case. You want to make them feel seen and heard. Hold their eye contact as you speak to them and let them know you take them seriously.

It goes without saying that your good bedside manner should extend beyond your patient and to their family as well. They are also scared and need the same respect and understanding that you show your patient. If you keep practicing your bedside manner, you will quickly see the difference it makes in your patient interaction and the trust that your patients place in you.

HOW TO HANDLE THE WORKPLACE BULLY

Everyone wants to be treated the right way. And while the saying is true that we should treat others how we want to be treated, the truth is that we teach others how to treat us.

Three years ago, I graduated with a psychology degree in hand. It wasn't long before I was offered a job at an institution that worked with autistic patients and those with developmental delays. Many of the patients seen at this institution displayed issues like aggression, extreme irritation and aggravation, self-harm issues, and a host of other maladaptive behaviors.

I was fresh on the scene, and I had a big job ahead of me. I was responsible for teaching these patients better behaviors to replace their previous unacceptable behaviors. Ultimately, they were supposed to learn how to integrate and behave in a socially acceptable manner. Most of our patients were sent to us by families who couldn't manage their disruptive behavior.

The institution I worked at provided me with extra training and education to accompany my psychology degree so that I could best help my patients.

I quickly realized that many of these patients were seen as bullies. They pushed every button the staff had—really, they pushed any button of anyone they deemed an authority figure.

I share this portion of my background not to boast, but to pass along some key insights that I learned and honed in that setting. After dealing with these types of clients day-in and day-out, I learned that the biggest factor in dealing with difficult people, including bullies, is in how you present yourself.

In other words, you must be the rock in the situation. Nothing the bully says can phase you. You maintain your professional, pleasant demeanor that you came to work with. You are not going to give anyone the power to change how your day goes. If the bully can anger you, he or she can control and manipulate you.

This bully should barely be a blip on your radar, insofar as the importance you place on him or her. If this toxic individual thinks that they are getting under your skin, you are playing into their hands. Do not let this happen.

So, what do you do about the bully in the workplace? It's inevitable that you will find a bully in one way or another. You might have a particularly difficult patient that loves to rile you up and pushes buttons you didn't know existed. You might find yourself bullied by those you work with or even a superior.

These instances can be frustrating, and you will most likely be tempted to return their bullying in kind. However, through my years at the institution, I learned that the best thing you can do for yourself is not to stoop to your bully's level.

Your bullies find joy in manipulating your emotions and expressions. That's why they poke at you until you react the exact way that they want you to. However, nurses are smarter than that. You are smarter than that, and you don't need to engage in any of the games these bullies try to play with you.

In fact, if you do partake in their game, you should change the rules. Don't play by the bully's rules.

Adapt the game so that you are the one in control, and you don't let the bully have the upper hand.

We are going to operate on our terms, not by some jerk's. This one point alone is the foundation for dealing with bullies. Do not react to their metaphorical pokes and prods. ACT on your terms.

As tempting as you might find it to return a snide remark with a snide remark, keeping your "poker face" about you is your best bet. Why does a bully torment you? They do it to get a reaction from you. When you remove the reaction they are seeking, the interaction no longer becomes joyful for them. They no longer find pleasure in teasing you or pushing your buttons.

You can't handle someone in your workplace the same way that you would handle them in your private life. The same goes for bullies. You can't pull up your sleeves and throw a good right hook to your bully in the workplace or participate in the backbiting they are baiting you into.

There are consequences for such behavior in the workplace. You don't want to be the person on the receiving end of those consequences, so don't get caught up in their negative behavior. In order to combat your bullies at work—both patients and other staff members—try to practice these tips:

- Always exemplify good conduct yourself. Don't allow anyone to point the finger at you and say you participated as well. If you don't gossip about other members and put other people down, then your own shirt is clean. Allow the bully to make a fool of themselves alone. In this instance, you will kill your bully with kindness.
- Familiarize yourself with hospital protocol and your avenue to make a complaint about bullying. It can be intimidating when the person bullying you is your boss or manager, but remember there is always someone above them that they are required to answer to. If you know your rights for reporting, make sure you report inappropriate behavior.
- If a bully gets out of hand, don't be afraid to document every instance. With this, you can show a pattern of their behavior. However, remember to not participate back in the bullying or goad them into being mean to you.
- Always be an ally to those being bullied. If it is your patient, you are their advocate; you need to use your voice to protect them. If another nurse is being bullied, be an ally to them and help them through this time. This

will create solidarity in the workplace that bullying won't be tolerated.

As you navigate through the workplace, remember that there will be times you are offered constructive criticism. This isn't meant to injure you or cause you harm. Take the criticism for what it is and don't inflate the issue if there is none.

MANAGING THE PERFECT PATIENT

Managing that perfect patient is fairly easy.

These are the patients we all love. The ones that are kind, know what they want, and clearly voice their concerns. They don't give us a hard time, and they always have a smile on their face.

While I don't have a lot to say about managing the perfect patient—since they rarely complain anyway—I do want to add in a note of caution here. Simply because a patient seems perky and happy doesn't mean that we should overlook them or pay less attention to them.

Remember your bedside manner when you interact with these patients and ask them all the necessary questions you require. Sometimes patients might appear overly happy and complacent when, in fact, they are hiding their true symptoms, and you want to make sure that you are hearing all their complaints.

Your good bedside manner will make them feel like they can trust you, and once you earn your patient's trust, your job becomes a lot easier.

HANDLING PATIENTS GOING THROUGH HARD TIMES

Inevitably when you work in the medical field, you will encounter patients that go through painful and difficult times. This might make them act out against you, and they might not be the peachy patient you want to deal with. However, they still require your utmost attention to detail and excellent medical care.

When you're dealing with a difficult patient or a patient who is struggling with a lot, remember to try and see things from their perspective. Are they angry? Are they yelling? Why are they yelling? When you put yourself in their shoes, you leave yourself an avenue to better understand their moods and actions. Allow them to express how they feel to you without you chastising them for their emotions.

Sometimes it seems like we're hitting it off the wrong way with our patients, and this can cause a frustrating moment or two. There's no shame in stopping the action, acknowledging that you two are not communicating effectively and then asking your patient to please explain themselves. Remember your bedside manner tips in this scenario. You might not always start out on the right foot with a patient, but you do have every chance to correct the interaction.

Showing your patient empathy is often the best route to relating to them. A difficult patient or a sad patient will be more receptive to your words and advice if they feel understood.

Sometimes patients act out in anger, and they will swear at you and hurl abuse. This doesn't mean you have to accept it; however, you should still treat them as your patient and show them respect. Calmly tell your patient you're there to help them, and you're going to give them a few minutes of privacy to compose themselves. Then when you re-enter the room, make sure that your body language and verbal cues communicate that you are attentive and ready to listen to them.

PROTECTING YOURSELF IN ALL SITUATIONS

Above all, you want to make sure you protect yourself and your job.

One of the biggest things that nurses can do to protect themselves when it comes to patient care is to chart EVERYTHING. Yes, I really mean everything. Your entries don't have to be long and drawn out. Just basic notes that get the point across are all you need for routine charting.

A medical malpractice judgment can seriously injure your career, and it can deeply affect your personal life. Your patients can easily create a suit against you or the hospital if they feel like a subpar standard of care caused an incident. This is why I stress the importance of listening to your patients and taking the time to sit with them and make sure their concerns are being addressed.

Don't skip out on taking their vitals and creating that connection with them. If your patients trust you, then they are far less likely to blame you if something goes wrong. If you've charted everything, then you have left yourself no place to be blamed. The three best tips for protecting yourself are:

- Document everything. If it wasn't charted, then it wasn't done. At least that is what the insurance investigators and lawyers are going to assume. Always chart what you are doing with or giving to the patient so that it reflects what really happened. Cliché, right? Maybe. I am quite sure you have heard this until you are tired of hearing it. But are you doing it? It's time to check in and make

dawg-on sure you are. If you find yourself sitting in the hot seat in court, this could very well be the thing that saves your hide.
- Make sure that you are in compliance with all medical procedures of the workplace. If you are in compliance and following the practice's procedures, then you are on the right path.

Make sure you're covered under some type of malpractice insurance. Some facilities have this insurance to protect their employees; however, you might still want to invest in your own malpractice insurance to make sure you are fully protected as a nurse.

If you are a male nurse like I am, always have a female chaperone when doing privacy-invasive tasks such as inserting Foley catheters on female patients. This is a practice I have always followed. It is just a smart thing to do. You just never know when a patient could have a beef with you and be looking for any way that they can get back at you, even if it means making up a lie.

A female patient that is angry at you for some reason (maybe you refused to bring her Ativan 45 minutes early...how dare you?) could very easily accuse you of touching her inappropriately. If that happens, what are you going to do? It would come down to your word versus hers if you did not have a female coworker in the room that could be a witness for you. Then it is 50-50.

It could end up going either way, and if you are found to be at fault, welcome to the unemployment line. And maybe a cell. Don't take chances. Protect yourself by having a female chaperone with you for these types of procedures. Not only does this protect you, it also is overall more professional and will likely put your patient more at ease as well.

INNER STRENGTH

Let's take a page out of the Navy Seal playbook here, one of America's elite military forces. Becoming a Seal requires enormous inner strength; but as the Navy knows, human beings are usually capable of far more than they think. Their training seeks to unlock this inner strength, and we can leverage this approach for ourselves.

We are going to dig deep within ourselves, find our inner strength, allow it to come to the surface, and shine it on the world. We have to really FEEL that strength, deep in our gut. The Seals have what they call the "40% Rule" (Myers, 2017). In a nutshell, this rule asserts that when a person's mind has convinced him or her that they can't possibly go any further, they are actually at only 40% of their true capacity. In other words, they have 60% capacity remaining that goes unused.

No longer will we face the world with a thin skin and allow every annoyance to affect our sense of inner peace. We must be strong. How do we maintain our inherent inner strength?

How do we get back in touch with it if it has been collecting proverbial dust since we haven't used it in so long? It goes back to our psychology. Every day, without fail, we need to work on building our psychology of strength. It is already there, perhaps some of us have simply covered it with layers of doubt.

A simple way to work on this is to challenge yourself in some way, every day of your life. The challenge can be big or small. We want to move away from our comfort zone. If we remain in our comfort zone, we will never grow.

One example of how you can challenge yourself might be learning one new nursing fact a day. There is infinite material and room for growth with that one simple idea. The more we know, the more of an asset we are to our patients and employers. There are literally endless other ways you can challenge and push yourself every day, and this is the path for growth and positive change.

Do we still need to work on it on our days off? Yep. Remember, every day is connected. What we do today has a direct and profound impact on our tomorrow. If we can get the present right, tomorrow will go right. And if we can perpetually work to improve the present moment, so that we get better and better as human beings, we will create a landslide effect of positivity and empowerment.

We will grow day in and day out. You may recall the old wisdom, that is so true, if you are not growing, you are dying. There is no neutrality. We can't just coast along and remain the same. We are moving in one direction or the other. It is up to us to ensure we are continually making bits and pieces of progress and consistently propelling ourselves into new and greater territory.

INDULGE IN HUMOR

What do you find funny? Any particular comedian or comedienne, movie, or book? Any specific situation? Any individual? Whatever it is, take advantage of it. Laugh as much as you can.

The nursing profession is a very punishing one. There's just so much pressure every single day you walk into work. There are very few days when nurses can just punch in and have a stress-free experience. Usually, nurses have to deal with patients that have some very serious needs. And unfortunately, nurses aren't always going to be able to meet those needs accurately despite their best efforts and intentions. This can be a huge strain on a person's psyche and mental approach to doing good work. Sometimes, there is a need to turn to coping mechanisms to help deal with all of the pressure and stress. Often, nurses will turn to humor as a coping mechanism.

There are actually a number of benefits to having a sense of humor, not just in one's personal life, but also in one's professional life. Primarily, you can use humor as a way for you to avoid getting burned out with your job. Humor has a very powerful way of diffusing tension when you're stuck in high-pressure situations. Obviously, being a nurse, you are exposed to all sorts of tense situations every time you put on your scrubs. However, if you manage to inject more humor, you will find these moments of tension a lot more tolerable and manageable. And a byproduct of being less tense is you having lower stress and blood pressure. These are all great ingredients for helping you focus on your work and not on the stress that surrounds it.

Some nurses might even be able to inject some light doses of humor into their dealings with patients as well. Granted, certain policies and boundaries must be upheld when it comes to establishing relationships with patients. More than anything, a nurse must always maintain a sense of professionalism in the workplace, especially when interacting with a patient and their families. However, that isn't to say that you shouldn't be completely devoid of humor when you talk to them. Part of having a good bedside manner is being able to treat your patient with a soft and delicate emotional touch. Sometimes, this means being able to joke with them every so often. Keep in mind that a patient and their families are also going through a lot of stress by being in a hospital too. They might appreciate having a nurse with a positive disposition and a good sense of humor.

FAITH

> Fair warning: If you are easily offended by Christianity, you may want to skip this section. Your choice.

I also have to touch on my faith in this discussion on maintaining mental calmness and peace. I am not here to tell anyone what to believe. The reader has the freedom to choose his or her own beliefs. But I will unapologetically share my own beliefs and how they are my ultimate foundation. Without my faith, there are countless times in my life where I don't believe I would have made it.

My faith is what truly keeps me together underneath all of my faults, foibles, weaknesses, and fears. It is what keeps me from coming unglued. What would I have done when I was caring for my beloved mother, who was fighting cancer, and ultimately passed away, had it not been for my faith? I do not know.

I am grateful that I did have a source of strength beyond just me in a situation in which my reality consisted of staring at my worst nightmare in the eyes every day of her illness. In Christ, we have infinite strength to draw upon.

You see, because of my faith in Christ, I view everything in this world as temporary. As long as we are in this world, we are subject to its ways. We are subject to disease and infirmity, hardships, and heartbreak.

That is the reality of living in this world, which Christ forewarned us thousands of years ago in John 16:33 - "In this world, you will have trouble." However, we are also promised that we will inherit the gift of eternal life if we accept Christ as our savior. When I think of life in the context of eternity, it produces a radically different outlook on life's challenges.

SELF-COMPASSION

When you're a nurse, you put a lot of pressure on yourself to succeed at work. Of course, it's a literal matter of life and death with your job. One false move, and you could potentially cost people their lives. That's a lot of pressure you have to bear on a daily basis. No human being is perfect, no matter how much you may want to be. More than pressuring yourself to always be perfect, it's also important that you practice the art of self-compassion professionally.

When you take the time to forgive and nurture yourself, you are doing yourself a favor. Self-compassion is a great way to build your sense of self-esteem and can help you forge better relationships with yourself and those around you. One of the major benefits of consistently practicing self-compassion is that it helps lower the levels of stress and anxiety in your life. This means that you are less inclined to more serious mental health problems like chronic depression. If you are self-compassionate, then you have the ability to recognize your own suffering. This will, in turn, help you recognize the suffering that other people are feeling as well.

However, self-compassion isn't necessarily the most natural thing to people these days. In these modern times, people just have a tendency to put too much pressure on themselves to be or act a certain way. As a result, they don't really tolerate failure or mediocrity as much. Too much self-inflicted pressure can be very dangerous for a person's psyche. So, whenever you can, try to practice habits that will help build your sense of self-compassion. Here are a few things that you can try out for yourself.

PRACTICE SELF-ENCOURAGEMENT

In times when you just want to bang your head against the wall, resist that urge. All people make mistakes. So, don't beat yourself up over it. Instead, practice self-encouragement to try to build up your confidence.

DO RECREATIONAL ACTIVITIES

Never be shy about wanting to engage in occasional recreational activities. If you feel like unwinding and listening to some good music, do so. Go for long walks. Take some time to meditate. Do anything and everything that helps relax your soul.

WRITE YOUR FEELINGS DOWN HONESTLY

This is a practice that will help you stay more conscious of how you're feeling. Also, it will force you to be more honest about your emotions.

PRACTICE MINDFULNESS

Rather than trying to suppress whatever negative thoughts or feelings you have, try to be more mindful of them. You should learn to validate your feelings because they are a part of who you are.

MEDITATION

Meditation is simply too beneficial for us to pass up. The benefits are incredible, but let's dissect this proven procedure and make it practical to fit into our hectic lives.

I often had trouble finding a way to fit meditation into my life. I had read tons of studies and various author's takes on it, and I was sold on its merit. Its benefits are documented (Harvard, 2014) and include:

- Lower blood pressure
- Relief of depression and anxiety
- Pain reduction

- Improved creativity
- Enhanced intuition
- A better connection with your inner self

The problem, again, is fitting it in consistently. I have never liked the idea of trying to meditate during the main waking hours. I experimented with that and always found that once I sat down or laid down and got comfortable, momentum kicked in—but not to my favor. Instead of helping me, in this case, a form of negative momentum took effect, and once I got comfortable and still, I tended to stay there, wasting much of my day. What I had intended to be a five to ten-minute session of meditation all too often turned into a two- to three-hour nap. Don't let this happen to you. What I recommend is to make meditation a part of your bedtime ritual. I believe this is the ideal time to meditate for numerous reasons. For one thing, meditation helps you to relax and ease into sleep.

SIMPLE MEDITATION TECHNIQUE

Many variations of meditation are possible. Here is a very simple technique that will be easy to incorporate into your lifestyle:

- Lay down on your back in bed as you prepare for the night's sleep.

- Bring your attention to your breathing. You are going to take ten deep breaths consciously, but following a special pattern. For each breath, inhale for four seconds, slowly. Take the full four seconds. Do not rush. Count to yourself, one-one-thousand, two-one-thousand, etc.
- After you have completed the inhalation, you are going to now hold the breath for a full six seconds.
- Finally, you will exhale for a slow and full eight seconds. Do ten repetitions in this manner.
- This breathing procedure will engage your parasympathetic nervous system, helping your body and mind to relax.
- Once you have completed the breathing technique, begin to count in your mind, backward, from 150 to zero. The idea here is to crowd all other thoughts out of your mind by occupying it with your counting.
- If other thoughts interrupt your attempts at counting, as they inevitably will, just take notice of it. Then, gently redirect your thoughts back to your counting.
- Ideally, you will drift off to sleep before you reach zero. If not, you will have gotten in a healthy dose of meditation and breathing,

and you will certainly be calmer and more poised for sleep.

PETS (NOT YOUR SPOUSE)

Whether you're a nursing professional or not, there are plenty of upsides to having a pet at home. However, for a nurse, having a pet can be very therapeutic. Think about the nature of your profession. You go to work at your clinic or hospital, and you care for hundreds of patients over the course of a year. You do a lot of work to take care of these people, but you don't really get to establish emotional relationships with them. So, in essence, you're doing a lot of work, but you're not getting much emotional fulfillment from what you're doing. Of course, you're doing your job, and your patients aren't obligated to express their gratitude and appreciation for you in any way. Often, they might even express displeasure at how you're caring for them. Being a nurse can be such a thankless job sometimes. This is where having a pet at home can be very helpful.

When you have a pet, you are also in charge of taking care of that animal. Let's say you have a pet dog. You would have to feed that dog when it's hungry and take care of it when it's sick. You'll have to train them and pick up after them. It might seem like a lot of work, right? Why would you want to add any more additional stress to your life? Don't you already do that with your patients every day? Well, here's the difference. Your pet is someone you can have a real bond and emotional connection with. And that bond is going to help give you a sense of emotional fulfillment when you care for them. It's going to make you feel really great to know that there is someone in your home who appreciates all that you do for them. To you, a pet might just be a part of your world. But to your pet, you would be their whole world.

If you're still not convinced, here are a few other ways in which having a pet is beneficial to your life:

- They might help keep you active and fit. Naturally, you will have to walk your dog, and this physical activity might be good for your body too.
- They help you become less stressed with everything that's going on in your life. They are playful companions who always seem to espouse positivity.
- They help keep you safe. If you have a pet like a guard dog, then you have someone who is always going to have your back in threatening situations.

HOBBIES AND FREE TIME

Professionally we are nurses, which is rewarding in its own right, yet comes with its ups and downs, stresses, and frustrations. It is also inherently a demanding profession, mentally, physically, emotionally, as well as in terms of the time and energy it takes away from our other life pursuits. Does that mean we should never loosen up and "let our hair down"? Absolutely not. Quite the contrary.

In fact, doing so is an enormously important part of the equation. We need BALANCE in our lives. Put too much focus and energy into your career, for example, and other areas of your life begin to get neglected, and they suffer as a result. Can anyone relate to looking in the mirror one day and thinking, "what happened?"

If so, there is a good chance that other things were taking precedence over your physical health and fitness. And there is a very good chance this was no fault of your own. It is just reality. If we don't actively think about these things, they tend to get neglected. That's why this is a call to action to regularly check-in on how you are doing in the areas of your life that are important to you.

Hobbies that we enjoy help recharge us, are a

source of fun, and help us grow as people. They are also an outlet for our stresses.

A hobby is an activity or field of interest that you indulge in purely for pleasure or recreation. Essentially, it's the things that you like to do when you're not working. Some people enjoy physical hobbies like tennis, boxing, working out, yoga, and basketball, among others. Certain people might enjoy more artistic hobbies like writing, painting, singing, dancing, and whatnot. There is no shortage of hobbies out there in the world, and it's very important for people to have these hobbies outside of work. As a nurse, you are bombarded with all sorts of serious problems at your job. Having a hobby outside of work allows you to dedicate some time for yourself without the constraints of pressure or stress.

If you're still unconvinced, here are a few reasons as to why you should definitely be picking up a hobby outside of work:

- They help relieve stress.
- They encourage human interaction
- They help you build new skills

You should already be convinced that you need hobbies outside of your work. The problem now is you having to figure out what your hobby is going to be. If you don't really have any hobbies or interests just yet, then here are a few principles to keep in mind to help you figure out what kind of hobby you should be picking up:

DO SOMETHING THAT INTERESTS YOU

Obviously, a hobby wouldn't be all that fun if you weren't interested in it, right? It's important that whatever hobby you decide on is one that really piques your interests.

DO SOMETHING THAT CHALLENGES YOU

Another important principle you need to keep in mind is that your hobby should challenge you to a certain extent. Yes, you don't want any added stress or pressure to your life. But partaking in a challenging hobby just adds to the overall fulfillment that you feel after accomplishing something.

SET GOALS FOR YOURSELF

Sometimes, the best way to figure out what hobby is best for you is to figure out what your goals are. For example, if you are someone who wants to lose a little more weight, then maybe your hobby could be a sport like yoga or CrossFit. If you set a goal to improve your vocabulary, then maybe you could take up a hobby like reading. Tailor your hobbies around your goals, and it becomes a lot more fulfilling.

TRY MERGING YOUR GOALS IF POSSIBLE

For those of you that are interested in picking up another hobby, ballroom dancing is an excellent choice. It will serve triple duty as a hobby, source of exercise, and a social outlet. Talk about efficiency! This is an example of using our limited resources, namely time and energy, wisely. Let this concept inspire you to come up with your own ideas. The possibilities are limitless. Just remember the key concept—if you are going to devote yourself to a particular pursuit that is in line with your goals, find ways to get more "bang for your buck."

In other words, let's say three of your goals are to exercise consistently, spend time in nature regularly, and socialize often. Instead of attempting to pursue three separate activities to check off all of those boxes, why not find one activity that combines them all? That way, achieving your goals is now realistic.

If you had to go to three separate activities, that opens up a whole slew of additional burdens, like additional time required, possibly additional money, and the list goes on and on. If you know there is no way you can fit three separate activities into your week, find one activity that allows you to achieve multiple goals.

Assuming your goals were the ones I mentioned (exercise, spend time in nature, socialize), what activity might you come up with? Do some brainstorming. Just make sure that you're choosing to do something that you would love to enjoy doing and something that would meet the goals you set for yourself.

There is just something about connecting with nature that has a renewing effect on the human spirit. Whether it be a warm spring day with a crisp, cool breeze, or a day hiking in the wilderness, we should regularly spend time in nature. It will benefit our mental health profoundly. Even if you don't currently have a vacation planned, just spending some time in your backyard can be beneficial.

PHYSICAL HEALTH STRATEGIES

WATCH YOUR BACK

*Always check with your healthcare professional before beginning any new exercise program.

This chapter is all about back health. This is a huge issue for nurses. We find ourselves in some awkward postures quite often, sometimes while simultaneously bearing weight. Ever found yourself twisting and contorting in various ways to get a task done? I have. Things in the real world just don't always go ideally.

Did you know that nurses exceed construction workers in numbers of back injuries (Howlett, 2013)? That is a profound statistic. Why is this? It is because of the cumulative effect of our day to day duties on our backs. As we do our jobs, we often push and pull on patients, sometimes patients that outweigh us drastically.

Perhaps one day, we have to turn an immobile, obese patient to his side so that we can change the dressing on his sacral stage three decubitus ulcer. The next day we have to assist a patient with limited mobility out of bed and to the restroom. And on and on it goes, with various tasks we face on a daily basis.

We, nurses, improvise a lot, and we are good at it. Maybe we planned to have our 350-pound bedbound patient in the hospital bed to insert her NG tube, but upon entering her room, we see that physical therapy has put her up in the bedside chair. Oh, and our techs are on break, physical therapy is now nowhere to be found, and the lift is broken. Yeah, these types of scenarios happen.

So now we have our immobile 350-pound patient in a much less-than-ideal position as far as the ergonomics of our back, and we need to get this task done before our shift ends in thirty minutes so we don't have to dump it on the next shift. If she was in the hospital bed, we could have raised it up easily to a good working height, so we wouldn't have to lean over the bed, which is murder on our backs.

That is the type of thing that, over time, will contribute greatly to things like herniated discs. All of this wear and tear on our backs eventually leads to the big injury that really gets our attention.

In some cases, nurses suffer from acute back injuries on the job, where their back seems fine one moment, and the next moment something "pops," leaving the nurse with a serious injury like a herniated disc that now has to be dealt with, very likely for life in one way or another.

HERNIATED DISCS

Speaking of herniated discs, I personally know a thing or two about them. I suffered from one about seven years ago, and while I am now at probably 99% function, there is still, and probably always will be, that 1% lack of the function I used to have. This is a common injury that nurses are susceptible to.

At the time of my back injury, I worked a job that required manual lifting on pretty much a daily basis, and I also lifted heavy weights in the gym with movements like back squats and deadlifts. These two activities, over time, took their toll on my back.

I was actually in the gym when I felt the first sensation of "something isn't quite right" in my left leg, in the hamstring area. It was like a sharp, sudden pain in the leg. At the time, I had no idea it was a herniated disc.

For weeks, I treated it as a pulled hamstring, to no

avail. My doctor ordered an ultrasound to rule out DVT, which came back negative and put me on prednisone and a muscle relaxer, neither of which helped it get better.

I went back to my doctor a couple of weeks later, and he referred me to an orthopedic surgeon. In the interim, I was miserable. I am a runner, and I could not walk properly, much less run. I could not perform well at work. I tried various remedies and researched ad nauseam. Nothing helped it get better, and I was worried.

The orthopedic surgeon's staff did an extensive workup, including an MRI of the spine. After the exhaustive workup was done, the orthopedic surgeon met with me. He was a young Caucasian man likely in his late thirties to early forties, tall, slim, and donned glasses that made him look very intelligent.

There I was sitting in this orthopedic surgeon's office, on a perfectly good day. I could have been doing any of a host of other things that a 32-year-old man might want to be doing with his day off. But no, I was sitting and waiting.

Waiting has a way of making us worry, especially when we are faced with a situation like this. I will admit this whole deal had me worrying. What was my future going to look like? Was I going to be a cripple for the rest of my life? Was I going to have no choice but to let this guy wield his scalpel and carve on my back? Just as I was getting lost and almost buried in these thoughts, the surgeon knocked and walked into the room. Having already reviewed my MRI and his staff's notes, he got right down to business. I was all ears. When he opened his mouth, the following words came out: "you have a classic lumbar herniated disc." Boom. Those words hit me right in the gut.

When the surgeon uttered this diagnosis, it caught me by surprise. At that time in my life, I did not make the connection in my mind between a back injury and leg pain. But as the surgeon explained to me, the herniated lumbar disc was leaking its inner material, which was infringing on my sciatic nerve. My sciatic nerve was irritated, inflamed, and making me unbelievably miserable.

It severely limited my range of motion, made it difficult to find a comfortable sleep position, and caused boatloads of PAIN. So now I knew my diagnosis, and the herniated disc in my lumbar spine was the culprit behind my ongoing sciatica. Now that the surgeon had hit me with the diagnosis, I was feeling pretty grim.

The surgeon went on with, "you have three options." I'm thinking, *only THREE?* "You can do nothing, and it may eventually get better on its own, you can have a spinal steroid injection which may give some temporary relief, or you can have back surgery." The option of doing nothing was not music to my ears at all, so I threw it out. At this time, I was almost crippled, and I wanted to get better sooner rather than later.

He had a polite and easy-going manner and was not over-bearing at all. He didn't try to sway me one way or the other. However, when I replied, "I will look into other options and leave surgery on the table as an 'ace in the hole,'" he responded, "I would too."

My exhaustive research led me to the conclusion that there WERE alternative methods that were worth trying. A common theme was various types of stretching exercises, which I found difficult at the time because of pretty severe limitations in my range-of-motion. I also came across some unorthodox advice that perked up my listening ears.

There was information from multiple credible sources that was advising me to hang upside down to provide relief to, and ultimately to heal, my injured back. I uncovered a method of inverting using what was known as "gravity boots," and I was almost instantly repelled by that option.

I'm sure it worked for many people before inversion

tables were around, but I could just imagine getting stuck upside down with those boots, and possibly getting mistaken for a bat. Batman jokes aside, I was sold on the idea that inverting could help my back. I just didn't particularly like the gravity boot method.

But as I usually do, if at first I don't succeed, I try again. And in this case, trying again paid off for me in not only the avoidance of surgery, but also the almost complete restoration of my physical mobility, and the total eradication of my pain.

If you haven't caught my method yet, the key to my success here was the inversion table. During the acute phase of my back injury, I used the table aggressively. The inversion table and inversion therapy, in general, is an excellent tool to add to our arsenal in the quest for back health.

Inversion therapy has solid research behind it (Sekhon, 2019). Many chiropractors use it, albeit a quite expensive version. My purpose here is not to sell you on the idea of inversion therapy. My purpose is to sell you on the idea that alternative treatments ARE worth exploring. I will go over some here, and there are many more that you can investigate. Going outside of the traditional allopathic model is worth it if you feel that traditional medicine is not giving you the answers that you seek.

I feel that I should address those nurses that may be hesitant about the idea of "standing on your head." I get it. Your reservations are totally understandable. Please allow me to provide you with some answers to your concerns. One valid concern is that this table that allows you to invert could "break" while you are in the vulnerable upside-down position, leading to severe injury. Yes, I have had that same concern.

There are some companies that produce tables that are of what I would consider to be a subpar quality, and this includes the sturdiness of the unit. Some of the tables out there just don't feel sturdy, and I would not use them myself or recommend them. However, the specific brand I recommend, Teeter, is exceptionally well-made, sturdy as a tank, and honestly would not break unless you were trying to break it, as in throwing it off a balcony or the like. The Teeter is the only brand, at the time of this writing, that is FDA registered as a medical device.

Barring those types of antics, you don't have to worry about this breaking, so long as you do not exceed the recommended weight limit. If you happen to weigh more than the recommended maximum, you can use an alternative piece of equipment that is made by Teeter. This portable decompression device will provide traction to your spine and give similar benefits to inversion.

With this device, however, you don't have to hang upside-down. You simply lay on your back and apply traction with the device. This device, along with all my other recommendations, is listed in the appendix.

As with any type of physical exercise, be sure to check with your medical provider to be sure there is not a reason you should not engage in inversion.

There are some definite contraindications to inversion therapy (Broatch, 1982):

- Glaucoma, retinal detachment, conjunctivitis
- Hypertension
- Spinal injury, cerebral sclerosis, acutely swollen joints
- Heart or circulatory disorders
- Extreme obesity
- The use of anticoagulants (blood thinners), including high doses of aspirin
- Middle ear infection
- Hiatal hernia
- Recent stroke or transient ischemic attack
- Osteoporosis, recent unhealed fractures, medullary pins, and surgically implanted orthopedic supports

If you have any of these conditions, do not invert. Instead, you can use the portable Teeter decompression device that is mentioned above.

I am not promoting inversion as the be-all-end-all solution for back health. However, I do strongly believe in its efficacy. I suggest that you at least give it a try. Before investing in an inversion table, it would be a good idea to book a session with a chiropractor or physical therapist that does decompression therapy.

The method will be a bit different than how an inversion table works, but the principle of decompression is basically the same. That way, you will be able to judge if decompression is for you or not before putting your money on the line for an inversion table.

While I can tell you first-hand that the inversion table is tremendously helpful in the treatment of lumbar herniated discs, that is not to say that it should be used for all back conditions. Please consult with a chiropractor to be sure that decompression will be beneficial for you, and that no contraindications to inversion exist in your individual situation.

If you decide that inversion and decompression is not for you, no worries. Just pick another of these methods that you believe is most compatible with your needs and lifestyle, and get to it today!

Bottom line: If you have a lumbar herniated disc, I recommend exploring inversion further to see if it's a good fit for you. Check with your medical provider and/or your chiropractor. Inversion therapy has a lot of potentials to help you heal. If you don't have an injury, the inversion table can be used daily to help maintain spinal health. It can also be used after any activity that stresses your back. For instance, I still use it after weightlifting sessions.

INVERSION PLAN OF ACTION

So here is the plan. If you are currently having problems with your back, first go get checked out by a good chiropractor. Also, check in with your regular doctor, which I recommend doing regularly anyway.

When you are a beginner with the inversion table, and especially your first few times, I recommend having someone stand by and "spot" you, making sure you can come back to the upright position when you are ready. Once you learn how, it is easy, but it feels a little awkward at first and takes some getting used to.

In my own use of the inversion table, I choose to fully invert. However, you do not have to fully invert to get the benefits. In fact, the table I recommend comes with a safety strap, which limits the degree to which the table can invert. Inverting only 60 degrees will give you the decompression benefits.

This also ensures that you don't get "stuck" in the inverted position, because with the safety strap, you can invert only partially. This makes it much easier to return to the upright position.

If you decide to use an inversion table as part of your strategy, use the safety strap, at least while you are a beginner. You may decide to continue using it indefinitely, as you do not have to fully invert to get the spinal decompression benefits. After my lumbar herniated disc diagnosis, what I did was use the inversion table once daily in the acute phase of the injury. I inverted for about two minutes in total per session.

That would consist of inverting for one minute, coming back upright for about 30 seconds, then inverting for another minute. I did this aggressive therapy every day for about a year. After just a few days, I noticed that my back was improving. Within a few months, I was pretty much back to normal. I could walk normally again, I had most of my range of motion back, and I could even run again!

I continued with the aggressive protocol for a full year after my back was better to continue to support the healing process. To this day, I still use the inversion table regularly. Since I am not currently suffering from an acute injury, I do not use it on a daily basis anymore. Rather, I use it to decompress after exercise sessions, especially after weight lifting sessions. I can feel instant relief after using the table for just a minute or two.

While I do not believe an inversion table can totally heal an injury like a herniated disc, I can't argue with the results. By using the table, I was able to get to 99% of my pre-injury function, avoid surgery and hospitalization, and even get back to running.

Although inversion therapy did not totally erase the disc herniation injury and I still have back pains at times, I can deal with these with an inversion session, massage, warm baths, and specific stretches.

If a few-hundred-dollar piece of equipment that I only have to use for two minutes a day can stop me from walking around with a limp, experiencing excruciating pain if I move in just the "right way," and get me back to my physically capable status, I am ALL for it. Find me another therapy that can do that, and I'll reach deep in my pocket to pay you for it.

Does anyone you know already have an inversion table that you can try before you go out and buy one? This will help you determine if this particular tool is a good fit for you.

The first time you get on the inversion table, take it nice and easy. Go back just a few degrees, and notice how your back is feeling. Is it creating a pleasant stretching sensation? That is what you want. If in the unlikely event you experience pain or feel that something is not right, STOP. Again, this therapy is not appropriate for everyone. But then again it can make a real positive difference in a lot of people's lives.

If you have an acute lumbar herniated disc and your chiropractor has cleared you for inversion therapy, I recommend the following schedule:

- Invert for two minutes total daily.
- First, invert for one minute, then come back upright for thirty seconds to one minute.
- Then invert for another one minute.
- You can use the safety strap, which will limit the inversion to about 30 degrees. This is enough to decompress your spine. If you feel that full inversion is for you, just remove the strap and go for it.

If you do not have an acute lumbar herniated disc, but you still want to take advantage of the benefits of inversion, here are my recommendations:

- You can use the table daily if you like, but it's not necessary.

- You can just use it at times when you feel that your back has accumulated some stress and strain, such as after exercise sessions.
- I suggest inverting for one to two minutes in total per session.

PROACTIVE BACK HEALTH

As nurses, we need to be proactive in keeping our backs healthy. As I mentioned before, after a twelve-hour shift, we have likely sustained some stress on our backs, and we need to take the initiative to do something about it. Otherwise, these types of things accumulate over time, and before you know it, you find yourself with some type of back injury that takes you out of the game, or pain at the very least.

I should also mention that it's not just the nurse that works twelve-hour shifts that needs to regularly address back health. Most bedside nurses really need to make this a priority, as the job by its very nature puts us in a high-risk category for back injuries and dysfunctions.

I strongly recommend the integrative approach to back health. The allopathic model of medication and surgery has its place, and for many people, surgery is a necessity. Perhaps they have exhausted all other options without benefit, or their particular injury or condition is such that surgery is the only hope for improvement.

For general back health, and to build a stronger resistance to back injury, there are several things we can do:

- Regular massage therapy deserves a spot on your list:

  o It can be used as something to look forward to also. Massage can be a reward for completing your mini-goals, and it can help combat back pain.

- I highly recommend yoga for nurses:

  o If you don't have time to regularly attend classes, you could attend just a class or two. That way, you could learn some basic movements, and then practice at home to save time. Most yoga instructors are knowledgeable about poses that are particularly helpful for back problems, as well as preventing back problems. Ask your instructor for some tips on specific poses and stretches.

  o If you can manage to make time for some classes, but not all the scheduled classes, that may be another good option. You could attend just the occasional class if you enjoy the classes but don't have time to grace the studio with your presence every time the door is open. What about attending once a month or so? Could you fit that in? That way, you can practice the moves at home in between classes, and keep up your motivation by attending monthly and feeding off the energy of your instructor and classmates. If you do have the time and inclination to attend classes on a weekly basis, then, by all means, do so. This book, however, is geared toward finding ways to improvise and make things happen even though we are strapped for time.

- Let me also provide a brief refresher on the things that most nurses are already aware of:

    o We tend to be taught these things as part of the orientation process at a new job, or as part of ongoing job-sponsored training. We tend to sometimes hear these things but not pay much attention. And we get so busy on the job, that sometimes these things seem impossible to implement because they add time to our tasks.

- If anything is worth investing a little extra time in, it is protecting our backs. Take it from someone who used to ignore this advice and paid the price. If you work in an area like medical-surgical and your patients have hospital beds, USE the height adjustment feature to customize the height of the bed for you, so you work in the most ergonomically sound position possible. I have encountered some nurses that still don't implement these fundamentals. These little things really do make a difference. Raise that bed up to a comfortable working position for you when you are starting that IV! Yes, it takes a little extra time, but believe me, this is a case where taking the extra time is seriously important.

- If there is clutter in your work area that will force you to take on awkward postures when you are working with your patient, take the time to clear the clutter out of your way. It takes a few extra seconds, yes, but this is an investment in your longevity in nursing.

After all, a serious back injury can sideline you from the bedside permanently.

- Similarly, if you need to pull a patient up in bed or turn a patient, GET HELP. Please do not attempt to pull on the patient by yourself. Pulling on a patient that is essentially dead weight puts an enormous burden on your back. If you plan to continue being a nurse for a while, you're kind of going to need that back of yours, don't you think? These simple fundamentals should be practiced without compromise.

Taking this little extra time is not a waste. In fact, it is one of the wisest things you can possibly do as a nurse. We have already established that back injuries are a reality in our profession. They happen every day. Since the statistics are against us, we have to proactively fight to ensure we do not end up on that statistic list.

INSTANT RELIEF

Of the many different types of stretches that can ease your back pain, I have found one type that is the undisputed champion. This will reduce like 90% of people's back pain. I have been thrilled with this, as it has an almost magical ability to put an abrupt halt to my achy back. Sometimes I still get back pain, which is mostly related to certain activities I engage in. For instance, after some heavy weight workouts, I may find that I pushed it a little harder than I should have, and now my back is fussing at me. In those cases, I will do three to five sets of this stretch, and I kid you not, my back pain is gone.

Of course, this does not correct any underlying problems, but it is fantastic if you are simply looking for some relief. The stretch I am referring to is the hip flexor stretch. In the majority of people, this muscle group is tight and contributes to our back pain. There are a variety of ways to stretch the hip flexors, but I am going to describe the most effective variation I have found. Even with a pre-existing herniated disc injury, this stretch never fails to give me fast relief when I experience back pain.

Here's how to perform the stretch:

- You will need an elevated surface in which you can lay down on your back. The surface you use needs to enable you to hang one leg off the side.
- A weightlifting bench is ideal for this. The bench I recommend in the appendix, while somewhat pricey, will last a lifetime and can serve double-duty for this purpose.

- Once you are on the bench on your back, bring one knee up to your chest and hold it there with both hands. Pull the knee as close to your chest as possible. Allow the opposite leg to hang off the side of the bench. Let the leg hang and relax.
- You want to feel a good stretch in your hip flexor, which is located in your groin area. Hold the stretch for thirty seconds, then switch sides. Do five repetitions with each leg, then take note of the relief in your back.

WORKOUTS FOR THE TIME-IMPAIRED NURSE

*Always check with your healthcare professional before beginning any new exercise program.

Let's look at the exercise component of our lifestyle at this time. With our notoriously long work hours, the drive to and from work, as well as all of our commitments and responsibilities at home, finding the time to exercise consistently can be a daunting prospect.

I believe that most of us understand the importance of exercise and that I don't need to sell you on that concept. However, many of you may know you should, and even want to, you just have not been able to fit it in. Up until now.

At one of the hospitals that I was employed at, I worked on the sixth floor. I made it a point to take the stairs every day at lunch. Our cafeteria was on the ground floor. But even if it was a day when I brought my own lunch, I still made this "stair excursion" on my lunch break. Not only did it release stress and tension, it helped keep me in shape.

I would take the stairs down to the cafeteria, get my lunch, and walk back up the six flights of stairs with my lunch in hand. Keep in mind that we do already take many steps as nurses, so our bodies are used to that kind of movement. It takes something above and beyond what our bodies are used to in order to improve our fitness.

Granted, taking the stairs takes a few extra minutes from your lunch break, but it is a very efficient means of getting in some exercise. Some of my readers may be resistant to the idea of walking up six flights of stairs on a regular basis. I get it. Perhaps you are not in shape for that yet, or you have any number of other reservations.

If you don't want to commit to taking six flights of stairs, could you take three flights? One flight? You have to start somewhere, and you can progress once the habit is established. Take a look at your personal situation, and do what works for you. The point is, there are ways to fit exercise into our existing daily routines. Every bit helps. The stairs thing is just one example. There are infinite possibilities out there. I suggest you take a look at your life and your daily routine and see where you can fit in a "mini-workout."

We also need a formal exercise program that we schedule ourselves to do throughout the week. I will present a well-rounded routine that is geared toward the nurse that is looking to maintain health, enhance fitness level, and become resistant to disease. This routine is not meant specifically to lose weight or build muscle, although it will help in those areas. The routine I will lay out has components of strength, cardio, and flexibility.

I don't have to tell you about the benefits of exercise. Let me just weigh in on this by stating that the benefits are very real. It can help you live longer and better, resist disease, optimize your mental and emotional health, and overall make your life BETTER. You will feel better consistently, leading to better productivity in all areas of your life. We are nurses, and we know the importance of exercise. **Let's bring it back into our lives in a big way.**

To consistently exercise, we have to make it practical. One part of making it practical is the time involved. I am going to provide options for workouts under fifteen minutes long. Now one of your biggest excuses is wiped off the face of the earth. Made totally moot. Even on a day when you are so busy that you can't even distinguish between the ground and the sky, you can get in a five-minute session. In so doing, your health will flourish.

Something about working out sort of "resets" us, both physically and mentally. After a stressful day of work, I found that a one-mile jog can wipe all that bad energy away and make me feel like a brand-new man. That is why I suggest doing your primary workout AFTER work. If it is your off day, you still might want to do your workout toward the end of your day to release any pent-up stress.

I should note that although working out later in the day is generally better for the reasons I mentioned, you also don't want to exercise too close to bedtime if it disturbs your sleep. Some people may find that the stimulation from exercise contributes to insomnia if done within an hour or two of bedtime. If it doesn't bother your sleep, then fine. Just something to consider as you plan your exercise routine and form your healthy habits.

HOME GYM

Working out at home can save you time and money. You avoid the drive to the gym and the monthly gym dues. Ultimately, your choice of where to workout will depend on your personal preference.

Some people find more motivation in working out in a commercial gym environment. If so, that is perfectly fine. The option that works best for your personal situation is what you should choose.

My personal home gym is fairly elaborate because I regularly lift heavy weights as part of my program. However, for the purposes of the program in this book, all you really need is a fairly thick mat, a pair of dumbbells, an ab wheel roller, a bench, and a swiss ball or back squat wall roller. You will find my recommendations for each of these items in the appendix. The options I recommend have been carefully selected and are used by myself, but feel free to also explore options on your own or use equipment that you may already have. If you use a commercial gym, you will also have plenty of options.

If you happen to have an extra bedroom in your home, as I do, that makes an excellent room to be your home gym. My extra bedroom actually doubles as a storage room and my gym. My strategic planning has allowed me to pack a lot into this small room and still have plenty of room to exercise, and I plan to reveal these methods to you in a future book.

If you don't have the luxury of an extra bedroom, there are certainly other options. The exercise program promoted within the pages of this book does not require a lot of space, so you could perform it in almost any room of your house. Find an area of your house that works for you, provides for privacy if that is important to you, and so forth. However, I would refrain from using your bedroom because you want your bedroom to be associated with sleep, not with working out.

After you have exhausted all of the workouts I have included in this book, you can play with the variables yourself and continue to progress virtually indefinitely. You can adjust rest periods between sets, number of sets, amount of weight being lifted, and number of workouts per week.

HOW TO WORKOUT

Resistance training and cardio are two essential components that need to be included in our exercise program. The third essential element is flexibility training. We will hit all three of these elements with the program in this tome. My focus in creating this program was to help nurses fit in the exercise they need with minimal time investment. Although the time needed for this program is alarmingly low, don't let that fool you, my friends. This program will provide you with intensive and effective workouts. Your fitness level will improve. Your health will benefit. Your mood will get better.

You know, all those good things exercise does for us will become a reality in your life.

I am going to provide an option for beginners to start with, as well as an option for nurses that already have some fitness training "under their scrubs." The program can be tweaked as you progress, to make it more challenging, which will help to continually enhance your fitness level. When you get to a fitness level that you are happy with, you can do maintenance workouts to KEEP 'yo fit on.

To add cardio benefits to our resistance training, the workout is designed to be performed in a circuit format. This format will also tremendously reduce the amount of time the workout takes. I suggest doing the resistance circuit workout two to three days a week. Take one day per week off from working out. On the other days, you can do the quick cardio workouts that I will explain. This way, we are keeping up the habit and staying "in the groove" of exercising.

Remember, we truly are creatures of habit, trite as that statement may sound. If we goof off and start missing workouts, we are only reinforcing the behavior of MISSING workouts, and astronomically increasing the likelihood that our butts will stay glued to our furniture. We don't want that. That is the path to blimp-dom and laziness, not health and vitality. We ultimately have to make our own decision. Think of it as a fork in the road. You can take the road to the left or the road to the right. But the road you pick will make all the difference as to your destiny. Pick well.

To be super-efficient with our time, we are going to combine the resistance training element and the cardiovascular training element into one workout. This way, we take care of two of the important elements of exercise in a fast and effective manner. You will still have the flexibility element left to do. We will take care of the flexibility part after our main workout. Stretching will help us to "warm down" and is a pleasant way to end a workout.

Hot tip: I also want to touch on an important concept that you will always want to keep in mind in regards to exercise. It is very important that you do not skip too many days of exercise. Sure, you will inevitably miss workouts here and there. Please do everything in your power to keep this to a minimum, though. One instance I can think of immediately is when you are sick. If you are legitimately sick, then hold off on the exercise until you are healthy. Other than things like sickness that give you a legit reason not to exercise, I want to stress the importance of being consistent. Not only because getting results takes consistency, but there is also a somewhat unknown factor at play here.

My belief used to be that since I have exercised so much in the past, those benefits should stay with me going forward. I am specifically referring to the heart health benefits now. I have been a runner for years. So, according to my previous logic, I should reap heart health benefits from all those years of running, even if I quit exercising now, right? Wrong. As I have shared, I am a perpetual researcher.

I have stumbled upon some interesting research that completely shattered my previously held belief that since I have done so much cardio over the years, my heart will remain healthy even if I stop exercising. This research reveals that the heart-protective benefits of exercise will actually diminish if we cease exercising. Specifically, the cardioprotective benefits stay with us for nine days after we stop exercising, but by day eighteen, the benefits are gone! (Lennon, 2004). This is a genuine reason to stay consistent with your exercise.

THE NURSE WORKOUT

This section will explain how the circuit resistance training works. The resistance training exercises I am recommending will work all the major muscles, giving you a full-body workout. I have hand-picked these exercises for their practicality, effectiveness, and safety. If you are already an avid exerciser and you have other exercises that you like, that is perfectly fine. And for beginners that choose to use these exercises to start, just be aware that there are hundreds of different exercises out there that you can explore, should you ever become bored with these. My recommendations, however, will get you started on the right path.

> Your workouts should always begin with a brief warm-up. This gets our river of life (i.e., blood) flowing, prepares our muscles, tendons, and nerves for more intensive exercise, and reduces the chances of injury.

I have included a three-minute warm-up option in the videos, but there are endless possibilities for warm-ups. When you start your warm-up, this might also be a good time to fire up some motivational music. I also recommend having your filtered water available to sip on throughout the workout. After the warm-up, move into the first exercise. I suggest doing the harder exercises, such as squats, toward the beginning of the workout. If you were to do squats at the end, you would already be exhausted, and getting through the squats would be more difficult.

As with any physical exercise program, talk with your medical provider before commencing this program. Also, if you have an acute back injury, you should avoid all weight-bearing exercise until cleared by your medical provider.

I am going to recommend some specific exercises, as I believe they are ideal for nurses. They are back-friendly and technically simple. I will also include some hand-picked alternatives to my main recommendations for variety in your training. If you happen to already be experienced with exercise, by all means, feel free to use whatever exercises you like. The ones I have included are very good; however, you certainly do not have to limit yourself to these. There are hundreds of exercises out there that you can explore. I just wanted to give you some of the best in case you are new to exercise.

Collection of the best exercises for nurses with alternatives:

- For pectorals
  - **Dumbbell bench presses**
  - Incline dumbbell bench presses
  - Feet elevated pushups
  - Standard pushups
- For triceps
  - **Dumbbell close-grip bench presses**
  - Dumbbell skull crushers
- For quadriceps
  - **Dumbbell wall squats***
  - Reverse dumbbell lunges*
  - Air squats*
- For biceps
  - **Dumbbell curls (seated or standing)**
  - Dumbbell hammer curls (seated or standing)
- For deltoids
  - **Dumbbell overhead presses**
  - Dumbbell side lateral raises

- Dumbbell rear deltoid raises
- Overhead arm raises

- For back
  - **Prone dumbbell rows**
  - Dumbbell pullovers
  - Back extensions

- For abdominals
  - **Ab wheel rollouts****

- For hamstrings
  - **Exercise ball hamstring curls (with or without ankle weights)**

> Note: Exercises in bold text represent the eight primary exercises. These eight exercises will give you a full-body workout. The other exercises are alternatives.

* Squats are a superior exercise. Let's make them back-friendly, as well as user-friendly. Back squats are a technically complex exercise, and getting one little element of your form wrong increases your

PHYSICAL HEALTH STRATEGIES

chances for injury exponentially. I have discovered ways around these issues.

For the purposes of this book, which is promoting exercise with the goal of general health maintenance, squats can be done with our back against a wall. This pretty much eliminates the stress on our backs and allows us to focus totally on working the musculature of the legs. It also takes the technicality out of the exercise and makes it simple to perform.

For resistance, you can hold a dumbbell in each hand. You will need a means of "rolling" on the wall, and there are a couple of options here. One is to use a swiss ball between you and the wall, and this option works very well. Another option is to use a commercial device known as the SmithShaper, which you can find in the appendix.

For variety, I am also including a variation of squats called reverse dumbbell lunges. This variation is also back-friendly, more knee-friendly than forward lunges, and technically simple.

** For abdominal training, the ab wheel roller is an excellent choice. It is technically simple to do, so it is difficult to get this one wrong. It is very effective at strengthening your core. All you need is an ab wheel roller and a mat to go under your knees. Any time you work your abdominals, be sure to stretch your lower back afterward. Here is a YouTube clip of some good lower back stretches:

https://youtu.be/soa9oz3RTVo

> I have shot some exclusive videos that will explain to you how to perform each of these exercises. The video can be found at this special link, which leads to a private area on my website. This link is for readers of this book only. The password for the private videos is NURSEHABITS (all caps). To access this exclusive content:
>
> https://www.beausalts.com/book-resources/

For beginners:

- Do each exercise for 30 seconds. Use your timer. Do not rest between exercises.
- Once you have completed all the exercises, you have done one circuit.
- As a beginner, do **one to three** circuits in a workout.

- Rest 60 seconds between circuits.
- Do a brief warm-down after your workout, which can consist of some quick, gentle stretching and rehydration.

For intermediates:

- Do each exercise for 30 seconds. Use your timer. Do not rest between exercises.
- Once you have completed all the exercises, you have done one circuit.
- Do **four to five** circuits in a workout.
- Rest 60 seconds between circuits.
- Do a brief warm-down after your workout, which can consist of some quick, gentle stretching and rehydration.

For advanced trainers:

- Do each exercise for 30 seconds. Use your timer. Do not rest between exercises.
- Once you have completed all the exercises, you have done one circuit.
- Do **six to seven** circuits in a workout.
- Rest 60 seconds between circuits.
- Do a brief warm-down after your workout, which can consist of some quick, gentle stretching and rehydration.

> Get yourself some type of timer. Egg timers work good for this purpose, but pick whatever you prefer. You don't want to just estimate on these timeframes. You want to stay honest, so a timer is essential.

Once you have done this for a while and feel that you are ready to progress, cut your rest periods between circuits to 45 seconds (while still doing the exercises for 30 seconds). When you get to the point that you feel you are ready to progress again, cut your rest periods between circuits to 30 seconds. You can continue manipulating the variables like this to make your workouts harder. In addition to shortening the rest time between circuits, you can also INCREASE the amount to time you perform the exercises. I have started you out with the 30 second recommendation, but you can increase that to 45 seconds, then 60 seconds, and so on.

For beginners, when you are comfortable with this amount of work, and feel that you can do more, increase to two circuits per exercise. Then go to three circuits. As long as you want to enhance your physical fitness, you need to challenge your body in new ways.

If you are new to exercise or out of shape, you can get a lot of mileage out of the beginner recommendations. My recommendation is that you ease into this. Start out with low intensity, and gradually build it up as you feel your fitness improving. Baby steps. Your fitness level will increase, and you may decide to continue advancing your fitness by making the workouts more challenging.

Alternatively, you can just maintain your new and improved fitness by continuing with the beginner level workouts. It is all up to you and your goals. Just remember this rule of thumb: if you want to maintain your current fitness, continue workouts with the same level of challenge and intensity. *If you want to further enhance your fitness level, you have to strive to push yourself harder.*

As a beginner you can begin the workouts with 5-pound dumbbells. Once that becomes easy, you can advance to 10- pound dumbbells, then 15-pounds. You want to continue to challenge your body. Don't worry about becoming "bulky" if you are a woman. Due to your hormone profile, you are not going to become "bulky" by lifting weights (unless you also have a tendency to inject testosterone, in which case this workout is probably not for you).

I also want to point out that although I have provided you with some great workouts, this is only the tip of the iceberg. You will likely eventually find that you would like a new workout to "shake things up" and prevent boredom. There are so many options out there for working out. I will be discussing more about this in the future, and I encourage you to research on your own as well.

POST-WORKOUT STRETCHING

After the workout is the ideal time for getting in your flexibility training. Your muscles are already "warm" and less prone to injury form the stretching. Also, you will be doing double duty here. You will be getting in the flexibility portion of your exercise routine AND "cooling down" after your workout. Here is a YouTube video with a great routine:

https://www.youtube.com/watch?v=FlAvRcz0zuY

THE IMPOSSIBLY BUSY NURSE'S WORKOUT

For those times when you are so busy that it seems almost impossible to get in your workout, fear not, I have you covered. I am going to present you with a six-minute version. It is short but effective, and it will help you keep your exercise momentum going rather than skipping a workout altogether. This one does not require any equipment, so you can do it pretty much anywhere. It combines resistance training and cardio.

The resistance will come in the form of your own bodyweight, using calisthenic exercises. However, the calisthenics will be done in an intensive manner, so your heart rate will be significantly increased, and you will sweat. As always, you should do a brief warm-up before engaging in any exercise. Also, you can do your stretching after this workout.

Here are the three movements for this workout:

- Air squats
- Pushups
- Overhead arm raises**

Air squats involve doing squats with only your bodyweight. Here is a YouTube video with a demonstration:

https://youtu.be/LyidZ42Iy9Q

Pushups are a classic, time-tested upper-body exercise. Here is a YouTube video with the proper form:

https://youtu.be/H3M1JgdjgW8

How to perform the workout:

- Perform each exercise for twenty to thirty seconds, depending on your fitness level.
- **Do the exercises in HIIT fashion, meaning you have to work as hard as you can for the 30 seconds that you are performing an exercise**. As you likely know, HIIT is an acronym for High Intensity Interval Training. As the name implies, this workout is meant to be INTENSE. However, because of the very short time intervals, you should be able to bring the intensity.
- Rest for thirty seconds in between exercises.
- When you complete all three exercises, you have done one set. For this workout, perform **two** sets.
- If you do the exercises for thirty seconds and rest for thirty seconds in between exercises, the workout will take six minutes.
- If you start with twenty seconds, work toward improving your fitness so you can do thirty seconds.

Like I have already mentioned, you can also shorten the rest periods as you become more fit.

With this workout, you can be done in six minutes, then get on with your business...so now the excuse "I don't have time" is totally obsolete!

**To perform the overhead arm raises, simply

assume a starting position as if you were going to do dumbbell overhead presses, only without the dumbbells. Hold both arms in an "L" or 90-degree position out to your sides, with your palm facing forwards. Your fingers should point to the ceiling. From that starting position, simply extend your arms overhead, rapidly. Do not fully lock your elbow at the top of the movement, as that would cause undue stress on the joints. Perform this movement rapidly, in a "pumping" motion with your arms. With this movement, you are targeting the deltoids, and you will find that your deltoids get tired very quickly.

As a side note, keep in mind that bodyweight exercises like these are very versatile and can be done virtually anywhere. When you are traveling, for instance, you can still get in great workouts with zero equipment! Just use your own bodyweight for the resistance and do HIIT-style workouts.

CONSIDERATIONS FOR NIGHTSHIFT NURSES

For this subset of our population, I believe you must be especially proactive about your health, both physical and mental. For instance, studies show that shift workers may be at higher risk for cardiovascular disease (Mosendane, 2008).

Technically speaking, the duties and responsibilities

of a nurse are consistent regardless if there's daylight or not. However, there is no getting around the fact that there are certain challenges that working a night shift may pose. The workplace environment that comes with the night shift is definitely going to force some nurses to really adjust the way that they structure their daily routines. One could argue that the night shift's physical and mental demands might be significantly different than a day shift. So, given that, it's very important that you still practice healthy habits while you're working a night shift.

GET ENOUGH SLEEP

We've already covered how important sleep is to your emotional well-being. As you know, adequate sleep is also critical for your overall physical health. This is especially important when you're working the night shifts. With the way that society functions, it's not natural for people to be staying awake all night. However, you just have to pay attention to your body's circadian rhythms or natural body clock. If you know that you're working at night, make sure you get adequate sleep during the day.

MAKE HEALTHY NUTRITIONAL CHOICES

One of the best ways to make sure that you are still staying healthy despite irregular work schedules is to eat nutritious foods. Sometimes, it can get really tiring to have to think about what you're going to eat when you're just swamped with work. So, try to engage in meal planning instead. Try planning your meals for the whole week so that you no longer have to think about it when the time comes. This will also help you track your diet better.

TAKE TIME TO EXERCISE

Exercise is always going to be one of the most important things that you could integrate into your daily routine. It doesn't matter what kind of job you have. It's always important that you are able to dedicate at least 30 minutes to an hour every day, three to five days a week, just for exercise. Physical exercise is great because it helps trigger the release of endorphins in your body. These are happy hormones that can help you maintain a positive disposition. Also, regular exercise helps you become fitter and more energetic as well.

BOND WITH YOUR COLLEAGUES

Misery loves company, right? Well, sometimes, the best way to combat the misery and stress that comes with working the night shift is to bond with your workmates. It is very therapeutic to know that there are other people out there who are sharing your struggles with you. It's also going to help build a sense of camaraderie in the workplace, which could help make the night shift a lot more bearable as well.

MAINTAIN A HEALTHY LIFESTYLE OUTSIDE OF WORK

Whenever you're off work, and you have some extra time, make sure to do things that you enjoy. If you have certain hobbies and interests, then indulge in them. Spend time with your family and friends. Do things that have absolutely nothing to do with work. It's important that you are able to strike that division between your work life and your personal life. One shouldn't get in the way of the other.

MONITOR VITAMIN D LEVEL

I recommend keeping tabs on your serum vitamin D level for just about everyone, but especially for night workers. Due to your limited exposure to sunlight, you are especially vulnerable to deficiencies. If you find that you are low, check with your medical provider about the possibility of supplementation.

USE LIGHT THERAPY

Working at night can affect your mood for the worse. Depression can set in when you rarely get any sunshine. Light therapy can help combat this. It is a medically legitimate therapy used by psychiatrists for seasonal depression (Virk, 2009). Consider investing in one of these lamps and turning it on while you get ready for work, or whenever is most convenient for you. An excellent option is included in the appendix.

SNACK AND LUNCH OPTIONS

Please don't skip meals at work. Believe me, I know that is often easier said than done. However, as I always say, you cannot take care of anyone else if you don't take care of yourself first. If you skip meals, your blood glucose is going to tank, and you are going to feel tired, weak, and far from your best. You are going to be more likely to be cranky, more prone to mistakes, and just generally off of your "A" game.

I suggest doing all you can to ensure you take the full lunch break that is rightfully yours. If there are days where you absolutely can't, then at least take five minutes and have a snack. Don't shortchange yourself in this department.

A great snack option that I personally love is almonds. They are portable, have a superior nutrition profile, and they are delicious. They tend to be a bit pricey, but this is a wise use of your nutrition dollar. The best kinds from a health standpoint are raw, unsalted, unflavored almonds. The supermarket chain Publix has the best that I have found. The product is labeled under the Publix name, so it is store brand but very high quality. The best option is the one that says "raw" on the label.

Technically, they are not truly "raw" because that would indicate that no pasteurization had been done, and these are pasteurized. However, they are as close to raw as you will find without going to specialty stores, and for something so healthy, I am quite impressed at how much of a pleasure they are to eat.

Dark chocolate, in moderation, can also be a healthy yet mouth-watering snack. You want to look for a brand with **at least 70% cacao**. It has an antioxidant effect and is beneficial to the heart. Note that you don't want to go overboard with this. Even though it has health benefits, it still contains sugar and caffeine. Just be sure to practice moderation.

To get you started, I will provide one delicious, hearty, very versatile lunch option. This chili recipe is from my family's cookbook, and it is delicious. It can be frozen and used at a later date or can be eaten right away. You can simmer it on the stove or use the slow cooker. It is very practical to take this to work and heat up in the company microwave. If you don't like ground beef, there are MANY variations to chili out there, such as chicken chili, vegan chili, etc. Just do a simple internet search, and you will be greeted with thousands of options.

Chili recipe

1-1/2 pounds ground beef
½ pound ground pork sausage
2 medium onions, chopped
4 celery heart sticks, chopped
1 large can Bush's Chili beans, mild sauce
1 large can Hunt's diced tomato (not drained)
2 clove garlic, finely chopped
1 teaspoon sugar
1-1/2 tablespoons chili powder
Salt and pepper to taste
1 cup ketchup
1 teaspoon hot sauce (or to taste)

Brown meats – add onions and celery while browning – (drain off fat) – add all other ingredients – simmer 1 to 1-1/2 hours.

Enjoy!

We like to top our chili with Frito chips, shredded cheddar cheese, and sour cream, but these items are optional.

HYDRATION

Water is the superior choice for general hydration. We are nurses, so again, I don't have to convince you of this. We already know a million reasons we should, it's just a matter of doing it. For hydration, I highly recommend using a water filter as opposed to tap water, or even most bottled waters.

I have experimented with a couple of different water pitcher filters. I was not impressed at all with the Brita, which I found to be cheaply made and, in my opinion, did a subpar job of filtering the tap water. On the other hand, I am a huge fan of the Zero Water line of pitcher filters. The five-stage filters do a superior job of removing the "junk," and the water tastes very clean. I chill it, and it is wonderful. I take it to work in a Yeti tumbler and sip on it throughout the day.

Granted, these types of inexpensive, basic filters

do not remove ALL of the "bad stuff" found in tap water, but the water has much less of these undesirables in it than it would if you drank it straight "out da tap." Most of the products put out by Zero Water are well under one hundred dollars.

If you are so inclined, you can splurge on very expensive water filters, some of which will remove pretty much all the impurities. There are many options out there. However, I, for one, do not happen to have unlimited cash lying around on my floors at this time to purchase one of these puppies. Frankly, I am quite happy with the compromise of the affordable, yet high-quality Zero Water. This company gets the Beau Salts five-star endorsement medallion. ☺

You are probably all too familiar with the science behind water at this point. Water makes up 60% of the human body. When you're not making an effort to hydrate yourself throughout the day, you are also effectively limiting your body's capacity to regenerate new cells and help you recover from the strenuous nature of your job. Understandably, you are very busy as a nurse. There are so many things that you need to keep track of with your job that you might end up forgetting to regularly drink water throughout the day. This is a big mistake, and you need to make it a point to be a habitual water drinker.

To help you integrate hydration into your daily routine, make sure to drink a glass of water right when you wake up. Without realizing, you are losing a lot of water as you sleep. Even though you might be sleeping in a cold room, you are still perspiring. So, it's very important to replenish that lost water by hydrating right when you wake up. Then, make sure you drink a glass or two to accompany every meal that you have. If you have three meals a day, then that's already three to six glasses. Then, on top of that, you should also be drinking a glass of water in between every meal. Also, finish the day off with another glass of water right before you sleep. Obviously, you might need more or less water than that depending on the level of your physical activity.

CAFFEINE

As far as alternative beverages such as energy drinks, tea, or coffee, you should remember to keep these in moderation. Keep in mind that caffeine is actually a mild diuretic. Sometimes, energy drinks are packed with all sorts of sugars that aren't good for you. Also, the caffeine in tea and coffee might end up disrupting your sleeping patterns. In addition to that, you might experience a caffeine crash in the middle of your shift if you take it too early. If you're going to take caffeine, make sure that you do so in the middle of your shift so that it will help you power on until the end.

APPS

Apps like Bite Squad or Door Dash can also be very useful on occasion. Keep in mind that these services are expensive because they charge a delivery fee, and you are expected to tip the driver. They do have monthly subscriptions that will waive the delivery charge for a monthly fee. If you use the service very often, then that would definitely be the smart move to save you money.

These apps include a choice of many restaurants in your area, and you can find plenty of healthy choices. Keep in mind also that there are limitations to these services. For instance, they are location-dependent, so the availability will depend on where you live and work. The hours are limited, so if you work a night shift, it will likely not be an option.

ORGANIZATIONAL STRATEGIES

CAREER DEVELOPMENT

ON-THE-JOB ORGANIZATION

As it is with any modern professional in whatever industry, it's very important that you develop skills at being organized and structured. Being a nurse makes it very likely that you feel like you never have enough time in a day to get everything done. But here's a newsflash for you, everyone feels that way. It's all really just a matter of you adjusting your perspective and practicing good habits to help make you more organized and structured with the way that you do your work. After all, there's no way that you can magically add more hours to your day. So, rather than trying to grasp at the impossible, try readjusting your approach to the way that you work instead.

Sometimes, being organized at work is merely a matter of getting to the workplace extra early. When you're a nurse, you have to make it a point to prepare for your shift ahead of when it actually begins. This is why part of being organized means coming to work at least 15 minutes before the start of your shift. This way, you have a chance to settle in and prepare yourself for the shift that awaits you. If you're just walking through the hospital doors with two minutes left until the start of your shift, you're already lagging behind.

Also, you have to make it a point to prioritize your tasks accordingly. As a nurse, you often find yourself wearing multiple hats. And it can get overwhelming when you're trying to track all of your responsibilities at once. So, whenever you know that you have a task that you need to attend to, write it down. Organize your tasks accordingly so that when you're looking at them on paper, you know how you're going to structure your day. Now, how you tackle those tasks is entirely up to you. There are those who like to get easy tasks out of the way first. But there are those who immediately want to jump right into the most difficult ones. Just do whatever is best for you.

For me, sticky notes are a key part of being organized. I'm basically the king of sticky notes. I sometimes have them all over the place in my area.

To onlookers, it looks like a mess. To me, it makes perfect sense and ensures I do not forget anything. The point is not the sticky notes. That just happens to be the system that works for me. The point is to use whatever system that works for YOU to keep up with your responsibilities that inevitably come up throughout your shift.

You know how it goes. You need to remember to change that dressing before your patient is discharged. You need to remember to check with the doc because your patient insisted that his Percocet 5/325 is "not touching" his pain, and he would like it increased to 10/325. You need to remember to return another patient's daughter's call for an update. These are just three of the countless tasks that come up. They always do.

Many of the tasks that come up can't be attended to at that moment, and they have to be put on the back burner. After all, we are the masters of prioritization, right? It was virtually branded on our brains in school. If we don't keep track of them, we will very, very likely forget them.

Depending on what it was, forgetting may not be that big of a deal. But please always follow through on your word if at all possible, whether it be with your patients or their families. If you tell a family member that you will call back, please do so. Believe me, I know that is the last thing on our list of priorities many times, as we are often struggling just to deal with the patients in front of us right now. But keeping our word is a big part of our professionalism, and it builds trust with our patients, which is a vital part of their overall perception of us as nurses.

What I do is scribble down a note on my sticky note pad as soon as something comes up that I have to put off but fully intend to get back to. Dumping it down on paper reduces some of the mental burden of the task, though that burden is never fully erased for me until the task is done. Most importantly, writing it down ensures that I don't forget.

Juggling thirty tasks in your mind stresses you out, increases your chances of making errors, and pretty much guarantees that you are going to forget something. By "vomiting" it down on paper, you can forget about it, get on to your more pressing tasks, and revisit your notes when time allows.

This brings us to the last tip, which is for you to organize your breaks. You never want to get burned out. Think of your shifts as a marathon and not a sprint. It's important that you pace yourself accordingly. You don't want to keep working to the point where you're exhausted and become unproductive. However, you also don't want to be slacking off too much to the point where you aren't getting anything done. One effective practice would be for you to organize your breaks so that they are integrated into your schedule and aren't done sporadically.

HABITS

When it comes to habits, the reality is we simply do more of the things we have already done (or avoid the things we have already avoided). Similarly, we think more of the same thoughts that we have already thought. The stronger we reinforce that action or thought, the stronger the tendency to repeat it yet again. This principle is rooted in psychology (Gardner & Rebar, 2019), but we don't need to get too deep into the research rabbit hole to come away with a principle that will change our lives. This simple principle holds the key to our success. The principal can actually work against us, however, just as much as it can serve us. As an example, avoiding working out today makes it more likely you will avoid it again tomorrow.

Keep in mind that part of being an effective nurse means knowing how to manage your time properly. You should be able to turn yourself into a machine that is capable of performing a hundred tasks in a single go. However, it can be very hard to turn yourself into a machine when you're limited by your own human weaknesses. However, one of the best things that you can do is to incorporate healthy habits into your life so that your professional career will thrive. When you condition your mind and body to consistently practice good habits, you will become more efficient and effective with the way you work.

If you're looking for a general guide, here are some good habits that every effective nurse should look to incorporate into their daily professional lives:

1. Never take shortcuts with medical procedures. Remember that there is a reason for everything that you were taught when you were studying to become a nurse. Always take a structured and methodical approach to accomplishing tasks. This way, you minimize the chances of mistakes and become more efficient with your work in the long run.
2. Always look for new opportunities to grow. As a medical practitioner, you know that the medical industry is constantly changing and evolving. If you want to maintain your relevance in this industry, then you have to learn to grow and evolve along with it. So, try to make it a point to always study the newest developments in your field. This way, you are always competitive and relevant in your place of work.

3. Manage your schedule properly. If it's possible for you to really write down every single thing that you have to do in a day, then do it. This way, you would be able to keep a better track of your time, and you won't end up shortchanging any tasks that you need to accomplish.

4. Practice clear and proper communication. As a nurse, you work with all sorts of people every day. In your line of work, you have to talk with patients, doctors, medical technicians, janitors, and fellow nurses. Given that, it's always important that you practice proper communication skills. Always be clear and upfront with anything that you have to say. Also, be a good listener. Part of being a good communicator is also being able to hear other people out.

5. Set goals for yourself. Goals are great motivators for anyone to do good work. Your goals don't always have to be grand and lofty. They just have to be stimulating enough to challenge and motivate you to perform optimally at work every day.

MAINTAIN AND EXPAND YOUR KNOWLEDGE

As you are well aware, our profession presents us with an endless sea of information. The things we are taught in nursing school represent only a small fraction of the knowledge that is out there in the medical world. New medications are constantly hitting the market, and procedures we have grown accustomed to sometimes change. To be as valuable as we possibly can be for our patients, we need to take our education seriously. To that end, school is really only the beginning. Maintaining and expanding our knowledge should be something we regularly do as long as we are nurses. When I say maintaining our knowledge, I mean going back and reviewing notes from nursing school once or twice a year. If we don't remind ourselves on occasion, we will inevitably lose the ability to recall a lot of the things we have already learned.

Let's live up to our responsibilities of being professionals with the knowledge and skills that our patients depend on. Accomplishing this does not have to take much time or effort. Just a little studying here and there can make all the difference. Do you have a med you often give that you have never taken the time to research? Patients are bound to ask you questions about it. By taking 15 minutes to go online and read some credible articles and/or watch some medically accurate videos, you will feel confident that you "know your stuff." How do you know if an internet source is medically accurate? Look for websites that end in .org or .edu, and you will rarely go wrong. Websites that end in .com may or may not be accurate, so they are best avoided when you are doing this type of research. You can find credible videos on sites like YouTube as well. There are many physicians, nurses, and other healthcare professionals that put out educational videos.

I also highly encourage you to stay abreast of current issues and hot topics that are going on in your nursing specialty. Be prepared to rattle off a fast, intelligent, accurate answer to common questions that patients ask. When you have worked in a specialty area for a while, you will start to see patterns. I have found that there are common questions that patients repeatedly ask.

Of course, some patients will catch you by surprise with a question out of left field, in which case you can politely say, "let me finish my rounds, and I will get back to you so we can discuss that." In the meantime, you can do whatever research you need to do to give your patient a responsible, professional answer.

Let's use COVID-19 as an example because this is all over the news and on everyone's minds as I write this book. Imagine you have a newly diagnosed

COVID-19 patient, and he asks you to explain what this virus is doing to his body. What you DON'T want to have happen is to stare back at your patient with a "deer in headlights" look, because you haven't taken the time to learn the pathology behind this monster of a virus.

You want to be on top of your game. You want to respond decisively, "this virus enters the type II pneumocytes in the lungs. These are the lung cells that are responsible for producing surfactants. The virus replicates inside these cells, killing them. This, in turn, creates a huge inflammatory response. This inflammatory response causes the alveoli in the lungs to draw in fluid. What does that mean? You guessed it—pneumonia. But this pneumonia is viral, so antibiotics are off the table. The lungs basically become filled with fluid and can no longer properly exchange gases." When you have responses like this at the tip of your tongue, patients are going to feel confident that you are a knowledgeable and competent nurse. As a bonus, you will also feel very proud of yourself, and deservedly so.

While you are expanding and maintaining your knowledge, don't make the mistake of trying to learn it all at once. Make it a goal to learn at least one new thing every day and review at least one thing you already know every day—this will have a cumulative effect.

Avoid information overload. I can tell you from personal experience that it does not work. I would often become interested in a topic, and I would search hungrily for every available resource on that topic. Then before I finished consuming those resources, I would become interested in other topics and pile up additional resources for those topics, and this cycle repeated itself. I would constantly be collecting information, but rarely even reading the information I already had, much less using it. There are not enough hours in the day, nor months in a year, to do this. Find one good resource and COMPLETE it. Once that resource is fully leveraged, you can consider other resources, other authors, and other viewpoints on the same topic.

During my weightlifting workouts, I actually read e-books on my smartphone. I have the Kindle app on my phone, and I also have a free music app called Rock My Run, which is for Android, and I highly recommend it. Between sets of my weight training exercises, I get in some reading on my e-books. This works especially well for nonfiction. I have torn through countless books using this method, and again, it does not take time away from my day. Excellent use of time. The same technique could be used for articles, books, or videos on any number of nursing topics.

You can use this method in your own exercise

routine. Find the "downtime" in your workout, whether it is rest between sets, or whatever, and make use of that time. Even if it is one minute here and one minute there, it adds up, and you can get through book after book this way, as I have done.

Speaking of music and your workout routine, I believe music is essential to help light your inner fire and maintain it. The Rock My Run app has many different genres of music, and it is not just for runners. It has music that is suitable for many other forms of exercise as well, including weight training.

During your workday, you should strive to learn at least one new thing every day. As we as nurses know, the medical field sometimes seems like a bottomless pit with never-ending topics and subtopics to explore, as well as new developments, changes, and updates to established knowledge and procedure.

FINANCES

I wanted to include a heads-up for how nurses can become more organized with our finances. Thanks to modern technology, we can largely put this area of our lives on autopilot as well. The more repetitive things we can put on autopilot, the more time and energy we will have available for the things that are really important to us.

I recently discovered a certain type of credit card that earns me cashback on ALL my purchases. This is extra money coming in every single month that does not require any additional effort or time on my part. All I do is make purchases as I would anyway, and I usually end up with an extra twenty-five to forty dollars of spending money per month.

The card I use is the Amazon Prime Visa rewards card. You do have to be a member of Amazon Prime in order to obtain this card. The Amazon Prime membership currently costs $119 yearly ($59 yearly if you are a student), and is a fantastic value if you regularly shop on Amazon, because you get free two-day shipping on eligible purchases! If you don't regularly shop on Amazon (and why not?), you still get cashback on all purchases. When you purchase on Amazon, you get a 5% cashback. Purchases at other locations do not earn 5% back, but purchases like gasoline get 3% back, and some other purchases get 1% back. There are many other cashback cards available, but some of them have yearly fees. I compared them all and found the Amazon Prime card to be an outstanding choice. I am already a Prime member, which does require a yearly fee but saves me a lot of money on shipping.

If, for some reason, you are not an Amazon fan (dear me, I can't imagine), please at least research the other options for cashback cards. Each card has pros and cons, so pick the one that is right for you. This is a great way to add a steady trickle of income that you can use for some extra spending money or whatever your heart desires.

As nurses, we make pretty good money in comparison to a lot of other professions. We work hard for our money, and we need to find ways to make it go as far as it can. This is another area of our life that can be a source of stress, and we can benefit from automating our finances as much as possible.

We can also benefit from maximizing our income and reducing our expenses. Even though we make good money, it may seem that we don't, because we likely have bills that claim most of it. For some of us, routine bills may consume all of our salaries. This is another area in which I have done considerable research and experimentation.

Finding ways to save money is a significant first step in getting our finances in order and improving our money situation. Of course, if you regularly engage in "retail therapy" and buy things you probably don't need, you can use the section on overcoming addictions to help put your shopping habit to bed. We first have to plug the drain before we can start filling the tub, metaphorically speaking. Once we have shored up our impulsive spending, i.e., stopped wasting money, we can start setting things up to work in our favor.

My first suggestion is to open a savings account if you haven't already. Don't settle for just any savings account. Look for one with a good return of interest on your money. In my research, I have found that online savings accounts tend to pay better interest, and I went with an online account through HSBC. I am very happy with this company and this account, and I have been steadily drawing significant interest every single month.

Interest rates are always subject to fluctuate, but I have enjoyed a pretty consistent return of an average of 2% APR. Compare this to the average savings account that earns only about 0.09%. This interest is essentially free money because you are drawing this money simply for opening a savings account and depositing your savings.

Tip: Remember that you must pay taxes on the interest that your savings account draws each year.

I have one checking account and one savings account. I keep just enough money in the checking account to cover my routine bills and expenses. My paycheck is also directly deposited in this account. My checking account does not draw interest, although you can find checking accounts that do draw interest.

The idea of having multiple streams of income has been well established, and I am a big fan of that philosophy. Having a full-time day job (or night job for the night nurses) may be our primary source of income, but having additional sources is a really good idea.

The extra sources of income can finance things like vacations, hobbies, and other pursuits that you may find yourself longing for but currently putting off. After all, your full-time job salary likely goes to bill upkeep and other essentials, with only a small percentage (if any) left for other things. This is where pursuing supplemental sources of income can be beneficial.

FUEL

Gasoline is another necessary expense that we can tap into and save some money. I have an hour commute to and from work, and I find that many nurses I have worked with also have a commute. Even if you don't have a lengthy drive, you still have to purchase gas (unless you Flintstone it to work), so these insights will benefit you. I have found a free app that works really well and is saving me respectable money on gas.

This particular app is for Android, but if you have an iPhone, there are similar apps available on your app store. The name of the app I have been using and am thrilled with is GetUpside. The app finds participating gas stations in your area with GPS technology and tells you how much the savings is on that particular day. The amount of savings can vary fairly widely from day to day and from gas station to gas station.

In my area, the app points me to Shell stations, and I generally find that I get an average of eight cents per gallon back on 87 octane. By the way, if your vehicle owner's manual suggests that 87 octane is acceptable for your particular vehicle, I recommend using it to save even more money. For the longest time, I was dead-set against 87 octane, primarily because of the "horror stories" I had heard other people tell about it.

I have found these complaints to be completely unfounded. A few months ago, I read my vehicle owner's manual, and for my vehicle, 87 octane is actually PREFERRED and recommended by the manufacturer. Since then, I have been using the less-costly 87 octane. I have noticed absolutely no difference in my vehicle's performance or fuel economy, and have been saving money left and right. I recommend that you check your vehicle owner's manual and see what octane is recommended.

It is best to stick with the manufacturer's

recommendation, and for some vehicles, 87 octane may not be recommended. But if it is, this can really save you some significant green long-term.

The GetUpside app directs you to nearby participating gas stations, along with how much the discount is on that day at each station. The discounts are usually broken down by the type of gasoline, so 87 octane will have a certain discount amount, 89 octane will have a certain discount amount, and so on.

You then click on "claim this offer" in the app. At that point, you have a certain amount of time (around three hours) to go to the gas station and redeem the offer. If you don't go in that time window, that particular offer will expire and no longer be valid. When you arrive at the pump, you fill your tank as you normally would, and be sure to print your receipt when you are done.

Then take a picture of the receipt with your phone from within the app and simply click "upload." The receipt is then electronically sent to the company through the app. So with a few simple steps, the receipt is on its way to be processed.

If you sent a valid receipt and within the required timeframe, you will get an email in a few hours verifying your cashback. The email will tell you exactly how much cashback you earned with that purchase! As an example, just yesterday, I filled up my gas tank with 17.84 gallons, and I earned thirteen cents cash back per gallon. I got an email stating I earned $2.32 cashback!

Not bad for no effort on my part, and for doing a task that I would already have to do anyway. Once your balance reaches $10, you can cash out your balance. Another nice thing about this app is that it has many different gift card options to choose from, including Amazon (my favorite). You can also elect to redeem the balance to your PayPal account, or even have a check mailed. This is an easy way to establish an extra trickle of income that comes in on the regular.

RECURRENT CHORES – LAUNDRY EDITION

As nurses, we are busy people. We all have this cycle of never-ending chores we have to do. Am I right? These are essential things to get done, lest we want to eat on dirty dishes or navigate around piles of dirty laundry in our homes. So the fact that we have to do them is a given. And this is something we all have in common.

The thing is, these tasks require lifeblood, so to speak. They require time, energy, even money. They intrude on our other plans, as I am quite sure we would rather be lounging on a tropical beach than slaving over a dirty oven. There are a plethora of things we would rather be doing than spending our lives entrenched in these perpetual maintenance chores.

Yes, it is important that we do not neglect these tasks. They are extremely important. But what if we could use our noggins and find ways to streamline these tasks? What if we could find ways to put them on autopilot?

That way, the chores get done without a lot of fuss, and without a lot of time and energy expenditure. They become simple, and they get done without really having to think about it. Then our time and energy could be put toward pursuits that we really care about, that we really find important. I have discovered many methods to make these chores easier and less time-consuming. Let's explore some of these hacks, shall we?

In this first book, I am going to focus on the chore most of us love to hate—laundry. I first want to touch on how you store and transport your laundry. My house is small, and my space is limited, so I have to be creative and think outside the box as far as utilizing every inch of space I have. I suspect many of you can relate. I put quite a bit of thought into this and came up with a solution I am thrilled with.

STORE IT DIRTY

For years, the system I had been using was just taking up valuable space that I needed for other items. I turned this over and over in the rotisserie of my mind. My bathroom is small, and I need the floor space. What I came up with is to store my dirty towels and whites in a mesh hamper that HANGS UP HIGH ON THE BATHROOM WALL. I found the perfect mesh hamper for this, and I love it. I will point you to it in the appendix. I use it myself, and I am a raving fan of it. I think you will be too.

I like mesh in particular for dirty laundry storage because of the circulation it provides, and the resultant resistance to mildew and odors. I place all my whites that need to be washed into this mesh hamper that hangs up on my bathroom wall. It is a little bit of a reach to place the items in the hamper, but you can actually customize the height that you hang the hamper when you install it. And I like to think of it as playing basketball, as if I am shooting hoops with my laundry. Makes it fun.

Now you also have to consider the hook that you use to mount the hamper onto your wall because the hamper will get heavy when you fill it with laundry. I have also already found the perfect hook for this, so this will spare you the time and energy of having to search for one.

You can actually get hardware to install the hook into a stud OR drywall. I recommend using the stud option if you have the studs available at the location where you want to hang the hamper, but the hardware options for mounting the hook onto drywall are very sturdy as well. Here is a great article if you need help with installing the hook:

> https://www.rent.com/blog/wall-hanging-without-stud/

Once you have this set up, you will free up valuable floor space in your bathroom. I have found that my bathroom is the most convenient place to store my dirty whites because when I undress to shower, I can just toss the whites in there, and toss the dirty towels in after the shower. And I always separate my whites from my colors from the start, because I wash them separately, and this prevents having to separate them at wash time.

When the hamper is full, and it's time to wash the whites, this particular hamper makes it super fun! It has a zipper opening at the bottom. What I do is unzip the bottom and let the laundry drop into another mesh container I have for transporting the dirty laundry.

The beautiful thing about my transport hamper is that it has good storage capacity, it is mesh, very lightweight yet well-made and durable, and it FOLDS UP to a very small size for easy storage between washings. I love this thing! You will find this and all my other recommendations in the appendix.

Between washings, I simply fold it up so that it's about the size of a Tic-Tac (okay, exaggeration, really about the size of a frisbee), and I sit it out of the way on top of a cabinet. Super-efficient and small-space friendly! It is perfect for transporting the dirty laundry to the laundry room. It has handles that make it easy to carry, and it doesn't take up much space, so it is easy to navigate through doorways and other tight spaces.

Ok, now we have established a fantastic system for storing and transporting the dirty whites. This really does make a huge difference in the ease of doing this chore. If you just used any old clunky basket or container, they usually take up much of your valuable space when they are not in use, and they are more awkward to carry to and from the laundry room. And of course, this is easier on our nurse backs!

I include other whites in the same hamper with items like undershirts, white socks, and so forth. I wash all whites together, and then I wash the colors as a separate load. As a side note, towels can actually be re-used for two or three days. All you use them for is to dry off, and you are already clean.

Re-using the same towel for two or three days is a very smart way to reduce your washing. Another tip is to be sure you have enough towels and rags to last seven days. This way, towels will only have to be washed once a week.

For colors like jeans, polo shirts, colored socks, basically all my "wearing" clothes, I have a separate mesh hamper in my bedroom closet to collect these when they are dirty. This hamper is a little different from the other two I have already shared. In this case, I wanted a lower profile hamper that was not as tall as the one I use for dirty whites transport because it fits better on the floor in my closet underneath my hanging clothes.

This one is more of a square shape, does not stand as tall as the other hamper, and yet still holds an appreciable amount of laundry. It has convenient carrying handles, making it easy to carry it from your bedroom to your laundry room. And this hamper does not take up much space in the bottom of your closet.

I actually have two of them side-by-side on the floor in my closet, in two different colors. One is for my scrubs, of which I have a pair for every workday of the week, and the other is for "wearing" clothes.

I wash the scrubs separately, once a week. I recommend that you invest in a pair of scrubs for each workday of the week as well so that you only have to wash scrubs once weekly. If you can afford enough scrubs for two workweeks, this is ideal because your frequency of washing will be further reduced.

All of these tweaks to your laundry routine may seem minor, but believe me, they make a big difference. I actually LIKE carrying laundry in these things! This system will make things more efficient, and you can repeat it week after week without having to think about it.

STORE IT CLEAN

Once the laundry has been dried, it's time to take it out and put it away. There are some shortcuts here also, and these shortcuts really make a huge difference! The putting away bit was one of the most dreaded parts for me, and I have a hunch you may feel the same.

> Bonus tip: Don't forget to clean the dryer vent after your clothes dry! I forgot this once in college and guess what happened? The dryer overheated and essentially "burnt up," rendering it totally useless (other than for maybe a paperweight).

I have found a wonderful tote for transporting CLEAN laundry back from the dryer to the area you are going to store it. This one folds up nicely when not in use. If you can't tell already, I am a huge fan of items that fold up for easy, out-of-the-way storage when they are not in use. I am not a fan of standard laundry baskets, because they take up lots of space and are awkward to carry, especially when going through doorways or other close quarters.

This is a big area to look for hacks! For one thing, go ahead and take the items out of the dryer as soon as it stops and take care of putting them away. This way, you will minimize the amount of wrinkles you have to deal with. Put the clean and dry laundry in your basket or the tote that I recommend and carry it to your folding area.

Dump all the clean laundry onto your chosen

surface, whether that be your bed, the table I recommend and personally use (see the appendix), or whatever you have decided to use. Now we are going to get into race mode, so you might want your boogie shoes. We are going to take a figurative puff of "speed" here nurses and get this knocked out fast.

For remaining wrinkles in your "wearing" clothes, I advocate using a steamer instead of an iron and board. I find that a steamer is easier, more convenient, faster, a lot more fun, and still does a good job. I found one that I like that is small and portable, so it can easily be taken on your travels as well.

Once the steaming is done, it's time to put your laundry away. For nice items like polo shirts, I recommend using wooden hangers and hanging them in your closet. The wooden hangers help the shirt to keep its shape better, and hanging your nice clothes on hangers is the best method for keeping wrinkle formation to a minimum.

For jeans and t-shirts, I opt to fold these items and store them in my chest-of-drawers. For the storage of towels and rags, I have a designated closet in my hallway, and I recommend that you have a designated area for storing them also.

If you are doing your whites, once you dump them out, all your white socks will already be together, provided you are using the sock rings mentioned earlier. And if you are using the over-the-door shoe organizer with large pockets, it is a simple matter of taking the socks and placing them into the pockets. Just fold the pair of socks in half, put it in the shoe holder (or in a drawer), and you're done. This method in itself makes dealing with the socks much easier and quicker.

I keep my sock clips in a cup when not in use, so they don't get lost, and are easily accessible. I keep the cup on a shelf in my bathroom because the bathroom is where I remove socks. I take off the socks, put a clip on the pair, and toss the pair into my mesh laundry hamper. Simple as that. This way, I will save myself time when it comes to washing and putting away the socks. As for your other underwear, they can all be folded and put away in a drawer.

I know of a couple of fast options for t-shirts (whether undershirt or "wear" t-shirt). For one, you could invest in a t-shirt folder and use a tabletop like the fold-up table I recommend to quickly and neatly fold your t-shirts and then store them in a drawer. I store mine folded-up in my chest of drawers. If you are not a fan of a t-shirt folder, check out this YouTube video for a great method of quickly and neatly folding your t-shirts:

https://youtu.be/uz6rjbw0ZA0

For nice items like polo shirts and other items that I don't want to wrinkle at all, I hang them in the closet on wooden hangers. I find that folding jeans and placing them in a drawer works well, so that is what I recommend. They don't tend to wrinkle very bad if you fold them neatly.

For nicer pants like chinos, it really is 50-50 as to whether to hang them or fold them. They may wrinkle a little worse than jeans if you fold them and stow them away in a drawer, but not overly bad in my experience. And if they do, you can always get out your handy steamer again.

I personally choose to hang them in my closet, because I happen to have the closet space available. Not because I have a large closet (quite the contrary), but because I have arranged my whole "ecosystem" so strategically that all my space is maximized. But again, pants like khakis and chinos could are really up to you. For super nice pants like men's dress pants and women's equivalent, I definitely recommend hanging them up to keep them in the best possible condition.

Regarding scrubs, I have found folding them to be easier than hanging. Scrubs don't tend to wrinkle badly when folded neatly and put away.

I suggest that you work out your actual laundry schedule on an individual basis because only you know your schedule and where you can best fit it in. You can also decide if it will work best for you to do it all in the same day, or to do a little bit one day and another bit another day. Whatever you decide, just be strategic and purposeful about it. How can you make it more time-efficient, so that it does not interfere with your other activities?

REVISITING DELEGATION

In nursing school, we are taught all about delegation. Am I right? Delegation can definitely help you get things done, considering there is only one of you and all. Let's face it—with an "army" of helpers, we could focus on the things we do best and outsource the rest. How can we make use of the delegation principle in our personal lives? Do you have children? If so, there is one source right there.

Another option would be utilizing the services of a good housekeeper. This may not be for everyone, but it is most certainly worth considering. Not everyone can afford a housekeeper, but if you can, they can be worth their weight in gold. If you can't afford to have a housekeeper come weekly, what about biweekly? Monthly? Bi-monthly? Find a schedule and frequency that works for your situation and your budget.

Please take the time to find a housekeeper that you really "click with," that you can form a long-term relationship with, and that you can trust. It is a good idea to be home when the housekeeper visits because, unfortunately, today, it is rare to find someone we can trust to that level.

If you need to have the housekeeper work when you are away from home, you can always install cameras throughout the house to deter theft, and only turn the cameras on at the times you want, if you want privacy at other times.

Even if you only have a housekeeper visit quarterly, for some of us, that may be better than what we are currently doing. As we get busy and life "happens," sometimes we tend to neglect things like housework, and before we know it, the dust is ten inches thick, and we forget the color of our carpet due to all the clutter. Ideally, you will arrange to have your housekeeper visit on a weekly basis. This will keep your home in tip-top condition.

The environment we surround ourselves in does have an enormous impact on our mindset, and as they say, cleanliness is next to Godliness. If you find that you are consistently "intending" to do your housework, but it keeps getting pushed to "next week," please leverage the services of a housekeeper to "whip it into shape." Once this is done, it will be much more manageable for you to do a quick pass on the schedule of your choosing to keep it in shape, whether that be daily, weekly, or whatever works for you.

So in between your housekeeper's visits, you should do your own mini-passes to keep the place livable, and never allow it to get out of hand. Once it does get in a chaotic state, you will have to fight an uphill battle to make it presentable again.

If you have trouble finding a housekeeper, you can ask people you know for recommendations. There are also established companies out there that specialize in housekeeping.

Here is a photo of the dirty clothing hampers in the bottom of my closet. The blue one (on the left) is for scrubs, and the white one (on the right) is for "wearing clothes."

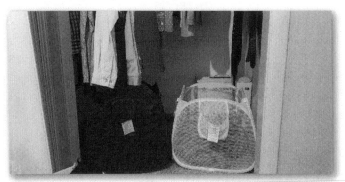

ORGANIZATIONAL STRATEGIES

This is the hang-up hamper for dirty whites on my bathroom wall. Notice the orange hook also.

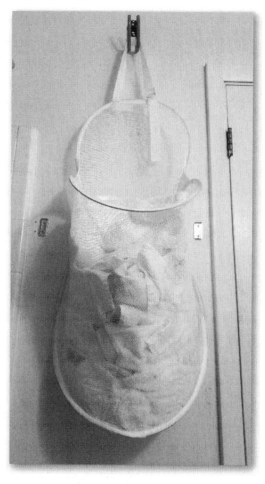

THE LOGISTICS OF LUNCH

We are now going to have a look at the bear of a chore that confronts all of us. What are we going to eat while at work? Some of you may already have a system that works well for you. A large portion of you, however, probably haven't quite fully figured this out yet. I know it took me a lot of thought, trial, and error. This section will cover some tips that will really help.

The best option from the standpoint of being able to control what you eat, as well as saving money, is to prepare and take your own foods. At least the majority of the time. It goes without saying that there can be times when you eat at your work's cafeteria or get fast food, or whatever else you decide on a particular day. It is a good idea, however, to have an overarching plan and strategy, and I believe that should be to take your own foods as the rule and do other things as exceptions.

If you have about three to five practical recipes or dishes that you love and can take to work, you will get a lot of mileage out of this. You want to have enough options that you have good variety. Whatever number of options it takes for you to feel like you are getting good variety is the number of options you want to have in your arsenal. If that number is more or less than three to five for you, that is totally fine.

Having great food and snacks for work is one thing. Having a simple, repeatable system for getting it to and from work every day is quite another. This seems to be the bit that most of the other nutrition books seem to forget about. For advice to be helpful, it must be PRACTICAL and SIMPLE.

The logistical part was the stumbling block for me for a long time. In other words, I might have leftovers or something I wanted to take to work, but figuring out how to get it there was a real pain. Complicated ideas just didn't fly in the real world. I finally nailed it and came up with real solutions.

After much deliberation and brainstorming in my own life, I have come up with workable solutions. Don't underestimate the value of a system in this area. Without a system, your consistency will be shaky at best. If there is one thing I have come to realize in life, it is that simplicity works.

Complex solutions to problems may look good on paper, but the implementation can be very difficult to do consistently. I believe in simple but effective, and I promote simple and effective, so simple and effective is what you will find here.

After experimentation with a variety of bags

and so forth, the best solution I have found is a BACKPACK. There is a specific backpack that I use and recommend. It is super lightweight, can be folded up small for storage, and has two large mesh pockets for bottle storage, which is super handy. You will find this backpack in the recommended resources and products.

The backpack frees up your hands so that you can carry your other nursing gear bag if you have one, or more easily carry your purse on your shoulder if you are a lady. Having your hands free from the burden of carrying your lunch bag just gives you more freedom of movement in general, and streamlines your lunch logistics.

As you know, hydration is super important. This backpack solution gives you a practical way to carry not just one, but two fluid containers. Maybe you have a need for two, such as one for coffee or a protein shake, and the other for your filtered water. Whatever the case, you will have the option to carry two bottles if you so choose.

The backpack I recommend is available in several colors, is very affordable, and is high quality and durable. Not to mention it looks stylish and cool. This backpack will enable you to transport your food, fluids, and snacks. This thing is legit! But wait, you say, the backpack is not insulated. What if you have cold foods? Enter my next recommendation.

The backpack is really just to simplify the transport. Inside the backpack, you will place your actual lunch bag, which is insulated. And yes, I have found one that perfectly fits inside this backpack and is large enough to fit a substantial amount of food and snacks.

I also recommend investing in several sets of travel silverware. This way, you do not constantly have to buy plasticware. And besides, plasticware simply does not do the job nearly as well. If you have seven sets of the travel silverware, you will only have to wash them about once per week.

You will also need a variety of containers. BPA free is always best for your health, and the brand I recommend is BPA free, microwave safe, and dishwasher safe. By the way, you should invest in a dishwasher if you don't already have one. This will simplify your life and save you SO much time. We want to put these types of recurring chores on autopilot as best we can so that we can spend our time on higher-leverage activities.

Isn't it easy when you have all the product research and trial already done for you? This will save you a lot of time searching physical stores and the internet for suitable gear!

For your water bottles, be sure to get BPA free. There is a hodgepodge of options out there. I will let you pick this one, as it's more of a personal thing. While you are at it, you should go ahead and get about three or four of these. That way, you only have to wash them every few days.

But pick one that is easy to clean, and that holds at least 32 ounces so you can stay hydrated throughout your shift with your filtered water. And select one with a good seal so you don't have leakage upon transport. Oh, and be sure it has good insulation so your water stays nice and cold throughout the shift. The recommended backpack easily accommodates my two large bottles.

The lunch bag I recommend also has a storage compartment on the front that is separate from the main large compartment. In this front pocket, you can fit your silverware, a napkin, and some of your snacks that don't need to be kept cool.

Once you have all this set up, you will be an armed and dangerously organized nurse! The headache of preparing your food, snacks, and beverages for transport to work is now simplified and solved!

AFTERWORD

I wanted to take a moment to genuinely thank you for taking the time to purchase and read my book. Mountains of effort have gone into ensuring that it contains value that will help make your life better.

Please do not hesitate to contact me if you have suggestions for future books, constructive criticism, feedback, praise, or anything else on your mind.

Author email:
admin@beausalts.com
Official Author website:
http://www.beausalts.com
Friend me on Facebook:
https://www.facebook.com/beau.salts
Like my Facebook author page:
https://www.facebook.com/AuthorBeauSalts/

**Sign up for my email list
and receive a free bonus report:**
https://mailchi.mp/984c5b627dda/
freebonusresource

DID YOU GET SOMETHING OUT OF THIS BOOK? PLEASE LEAVE A REVIEW ON AMAZON!

ABOUT THE AUTHOR

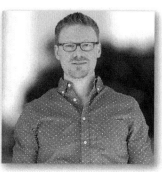

Beau Salts is a hard-working registered nurse full-time. He is interested in all topics medical-related, and in nursing school, his nose probably got tired of being glued to textbooks so often. Fortunately, his nose never complained.

Beau is physically active and loves dogs. He is all-American and loves southern food. Having always had a knack for writing, Beau is happy to be bringing his life lessons to the world through the written word. The Beau Salts brand is just getting started, and there is MUCH more to come!

APPENDIX 1:
RECOMMENDED PRODUCTS

Note: These are not affiliate links. I use and believe in these products. They are worth your time and investment.

1. Travel silverware (includes chopsticks, for you sophisticated nurses) HERE: https://beausalts.com/xyxh

2. Sock locks HERE: https://beausalts.com/7u5h

3. Blackout curtains HERE: https://beausalts.com/81rr

4. Portable steamer HERE: https://beausalts.com/c7u9

5. Fold-up table (great for folding laundry) HERE: https://beausalts.com/qvdb

6. Hook for laundry hamper HERE: https://beausalts.com/c1zs

7. Lunch bag HERE: https://beausalts.com/8wsl

8. Backpack HERE: https://beausalts.com/25l6

9. Hanging mesh hamper HERE: https://beausalts.com/lt9n

10. Over-the-door shoe organizer HERE: https://beausalts.com/bgdy

11. Square laundry hamper HERE: https://beausalts.com/fonl

12. Water tester HERE: https://beausalts.com/sgr8

13. Zero water filter pitcher HERE: https://beausalts.com/ldx5

14. Collapsible laundry tote HERE: https://beausalts.com/j7qi

15. Mesh laundry hamper (this is the one I recommend for transporting dirty whites to washing machine) HERE: https://beausalts.com/4ojy

16. Shirt folding board HERE: https://beausalts.com/isnl

17. Exercise mat (marketed as jump-rope mat but good for our exercise program) HERE: https://beausalts.com/1d91

18. Ab roller HERE:
    https://beausalts.com/tiiv

19. Essential oil diffuser HERE:
    https://beausalts.com/uyd7

20. Light therapy (recommended especially for night-shift nurses) HERE:
    https://beausalts.com/iap4

21. Blue-light glasses HERE:
    https://beausalts.com/m7qr

22. Wall squat roller HERE:
    https://beausalts.com/9i95

23. Exercise ball for wall squats HERE:
    https://beausalts.com/ynnj

24. Weight bench HERE:
    https://beausalts.com/bcvp

25. Adjustable ankle/wrist weights HERE:
    https://beausalts.com/joda

26. Inversion table HERE:
    https://beausalts.com/tfe0

27. Portable inversion unit (alternative to hanging upside-down) HERE:
    https://beausalts.com/nj0m

28. Therapy Putty HERE:
    https://beausalts.com/zuzu

APPENDIX 2:
RESOURCES BY CHAPTER

MENTAL STRATEGIES

Doheny, K. (2008). Can't Sleep? Adjust the Temperature. Retrieved from https://www.webmd.com/sleep-disorders/features/cant-sleep-adjust-the-temperature#1

EMOTIONAL STRATEGIES

Harvard Health Publishing. (2014). What Meditation can do for your Mind, Mood, and Health. Retrieved from https://www.health.harvard.edu/staying-healthy/what-meditation-can-do-for-your-mind-mood-and-health-

Myers, Chris. (2017). The 40% Rule: The Simple Secret to Success. Retrieved from
https://www.forbes.com/sites/chrismyers/2017/10/06/the-40-rule-the-simple-secret-to-success/

Lippincott Williams & Wilkins. (n.d.) How to Protect Yourself from Malpractice. Retrieved from
https://www.nursingcenter.com/upload/journals/documents/200303nsoce2protect.htm

Walker, A. (n.d.) 10 Tips for Dealing with Difficult Patients. Retrieved from
https://nurse.org/articles/dealing-with-difficult-patients/

PHYSICAL HEALTH STRATEGIES

Howlett, Hill. (2013). Success in Practical/Vocational Nursing: From Student to Leader.

Mosendane, Thabo MB ChB, et al. (2008). Shift Work and its Effects on the Cardiovascular System. Retrieved from
https://www.ncbi.nlm.nih.gov/pmc/articles/PMC3971766/

Virk, Gagan MD, et al. (2009). Short Exposure to Light Treatment Improves Depression Scores in Patients with Seasonal Affective Disorder: A Brief Report. Retrieved from https://www.ncbi.nlm.nih.gov/pmc/articles/PMC2913518/

Broatch, Joanne. (1982). Better Back Better Body: The New Inversion Way.

Sekhon, Lali MD PhD. (Updated 2019). Turning Back Pain and Sciatica Upside Down. Retrieved from https://www.spineuniverse.com/conditions/back-pain/low-back-pain/turning-back-pain-sciatica-upside-down

Lennon, Shannon, et al. (2004). Loss of Exercise-Induced Cardioprotection after Cessation of Exercise. Retrieved from https://journals.physiology.org/doi/full/10.1152/japplphysiol.00920.2003

ORGANIZATIONAL STRATEGIES

Gardner, B., & Rebar, A. (2019). Habit Formation and Behavior Change. Retrieved from https://oxfordre.com/psychology/view/10.1093/acrefore/9780190236557.001.0001/acrefore-9780190236557-e-129

Made in the USA
Monee, IL
18 June 2020